The Marlowe Diabetes Library
Good control is in your hands.

SINCE 1999, Marlowe & Company has established itself as the nation's leading independent publisher of books on diabetes. Now, the Marlowe Diabetes Library, launched in 2007, comprises an ever-expanding list of books on how to thrive while living with diabetes or prediabetes. Authors include world-renowned authorities on diabetes and the glycemic index, medical doctors and research scientists, certified diabetes educators, registered dietitians and other professional clinicians, as well as individuals living and thriving with prediabetes, type 1 or type 2 diabetes. See page 299 for the complete list of Marlowe Diabetes Library titles.

RICHARD JACKSON, MD, is currently Director of Outreach at the Joslin Diabetes Center, and Assistant Professor of Medicine at Harvard Medical School. In addition, Dr. Jackson is a Senior Investigator in the Research Division (Section on Immunology and Immunogenetics), where he established, and was the Director of the Hood Center for Prevention of Childhood Diabetes. He is also a member of the Joslin's Clinical Division, where he serves as Medical Director of the Joslin's Diabetes Outpatient Intensive Treatment (DOIT) Program. He is a former Mary K. Iacocca Fellow and recipient of the Cookie Pierce Research Award from the Juvenile Diabetes Research Foundation. He lives in Brookline, Massahcusetts.

AMY TENDERICH is a professional journalist with an MA in communication studies who was diagnosed with type 1 diabetes in May 2003 (in her mid-thirties). Almost instantly, she began to tell it like it is on her own diabetes blog (www.DiabetesMine.com), for which she recently received the LillyforLife Achievement Award for diabetes journalism. Tenderich now also brings her unique observations on the challenges of living with diabetes to *dLife* in a monthly column, and does double-duty as a full-time mom. She and her family live just south of San Francisco, California.

Richard Jackson, MD & Amy Tenderich

Know Your Numbers, Outlive Your Diabetes

**Five Essential
Health Factors
You Can Master
to Enjoy a Long
and Healthy Life**

MARLOWE & COMPANY
NEW YORK

KNOW YOUR NUMBERS, OUTLIVE YOUR DIABETES:
Five Essential Health Factors You Can Master to Enjoy a Long and Healthy Life

Copyright © 2007 Richard Jackson and Amy Tenderich

Published by
Marlowe & Company
An Imprint of Avalon Publishing Group, Incorporated
245 West 17th Street • 11th Floor
New York, NY 10011-5300

AVALON

Library of Congress Cataloging-in-Publication Data

Jackson, Richard (Richard Alan).
    Know your numbers, outlive your diabetes : five essential health factors you can master to enjoy a long and healthy life / [Richard Jackson and Amy Tenderich].
       p. cm.
    ISBN-13: 978-1-56924-272-8 (trade pbk.)
    ISBN-10: 1-56924-272-0 (trade pbk.)
    1. Diabetes—Popular works. 2. Health status indicators. I. Tenderich, Amy.
II. Title.
RC660.4.J33 2007
616.4'62—dc22

                                                                2006032669

The information in this book is intended to help readers make informed decisions about their health and the health of their loved ones. It is not intended to be a substitute for treatment by or the advice and care of a professional health-care provider. While the author and publisher have endeavored to ensure that the information presented is accurate and up to date, they are not responsible for adverse effects or consequences sustained by any person using this book.

9 8 7 6 5 4 3

DESIGNED BY PAULINE NEUWIRTH, NEUWIRTH & ASSOCIATES, INC.

Printed in the United States of America

This book is dedicated to:

Susan, who keeps me centered, and to all my patients, who have taught me so much.

—RICHARD JACKSON

My amazing husband, Burghardt, who encouraged me to turn my diabetes into something positive.

—AMY TENDERICH

Bill Polonsky, PhD, CDE, for caring enough about people's psychological struggles with diabetes to actually do something about it—and for bringing us together to make this long-imagined book happen.

—AMY AND RICH

Contents

Preface

WHY DID WE write this book?

Because so many people start off with the wrong ideas about diabetes, and they're quickly overwhelmed. They think they have to do everything at once (alter their diet, lose twenty pounds, start a rigorous exercise program, tighten their glucose control, etc.). But doing all that at once is just too difficult. And guess what? It doesn't even make sense from a health standpoint.

Often people focus on the stuff they feel guilty about (usually weight or food), when that may not even be their most critical health issue.

What people *don't* usually do is get the hard facts on where they stand in terms of their own diabetes health risks. They either haven't had the five essential diabetes health tests, or they have no idea what the results are or what they might mean. But these five tests—your A1c, blood pressure, lipids, microalbumin, and eye exam—provide the essential information you need to understand and manage your own health with diabetes.

Meanwhile, all of us want to live a long and healthy life, despite our diabetes. So the point we'll hammer home in this book is: *how can you get where you're going if don't know where you're starting from?*

We've seen this too often: people worrying that they need to drastically change their eating, and lose forty pounds, when maybe what they really need is a walking program and a blood pressure medication. Without *knowing their numbers*, they don't know where they are, and that naturally makes it difficult to reach their goal of outliving their diabetes.

Dr. Richard A. Jackson has helped thousands of people with type 2 diabetes from all over the country for over twenty years at Joslin Diabetes Center in Boston. He's an active researcher who's also taken a leading role in developing and implementing the Joslin "DO-IT" diabetes outpatient treatment program, the only personalized intensive diabetes management course of its kind.

Journalist Amy Tenderich was diagnosed with type 1 diabetes in 2003, and has since become a prominent voice in the diabetes community through her columns, articles, and Web site, www.diabetesmine.com.

That's who we are. And the reason we care is that we both know lots of people who have feelings, ideas, and opinions about their diabetes—but don't really know the actual status of their own health. Too often they focus in on one factor—it's all about the glucose readings, or all about the food—with constant frustration. But there is a better way. For the first time in history, the *specific* tools and knowledge you need to live long and well with diabetes are readily available. Consider this:

In the past, people were essentially groping in the dark with their diabetes. The tests and methods available were so primitive that it really was like fumbling in a dark room toward the door marked "Exit Here for a Long and Healthy Life" that you knew was there, but couldn't see. Since, for example, doctors could only guess at their daily glucose levels, patients were subjected to all sorts of drills—like eating the same bland food for dinner every night for years on end—in the hope that this would keep their diabetes in control.

But now the light in that dark room has been switched on. Improved laboratory tests and advanced tools such as home glucose meters let you see where you're going—and sometimes you'll find there are more paths than you realized that enable you to reach that same exit from the other side of room. You now have some flexibility in your health improvement choices.

This book will help walk you through three important certainties:

- It is vital to find out where you are with your diabetes, i.e., to know and understand your personal health/risk factors.
- You can and should prioritize your efforts, so you're only working on your own individual *one or two* key health efforts at a time.
- Your efforts (and not just your doctor's) make a significant difference in your health right now, and in achieving the long and healthy life you want.

We wrote this book to serve as a comprehensive, hands-on guide to successfully managing your own health.

How to Use This Book

BE AWARE THAT the first four chapters of this book are your
"action chapters"—offering the crux of *Know Your Numbers,
Outlive Your Diabetes* in a nutshell. Our goal is to offer you enough
information for you to start getting a handle on your health with diabetes right away, even if all you read are these first four chapters.

However, you'll find that there's a lot of useful information in the
rest of the book as well. Go ahead and skip to the chapters that
interest you most. It's probably well worth keeping this book in your
nightstand or otherwise close at hand as a quick reference guide
on all things diabetic.

Regarding Sources

AT TIMES, WE provide our thoughts on various matters related to
diabetes. We would like to make clear that we've formulated these
opinions based on our experience and knowledge, informed by
research, physiology, and critical discussion.

Therefore, the approaches and information presented in most

chapters are *not* simply our personal opinions, but rather the clear-cut, commonly accepted results of multiple clinical studies regarding the five core diabetes factors: your A1c, blood pressure, lipids, microalbumin, and eye exam.

The ★ in this book alerts to you to our specific recommendations, while the ■ highlights the backdrop for our choices, informed by the recommendations of other authorities.

Although there may be some disagreement about some of the recommendations we make in this book, there cannot be any disagreement about the very important basics of these five core tests and their significance to your health.

A Medication Disclaimer

WE DESCRIBE A number of medications in this book, to help you be better informed about your choices. However, do be sure to consult with your health-care provider before taking any of these drugs.

Notes on Blood Glucose Terminology

MANY PEOPLE TALK about "blood sugar"; the sugar present in your blood is *glucose*, the common fuel used by your body's cells for energy. Because there are many different sugars, and because glucose is more exact, we use the term *blood glucose* (BG) throughout this book.

In addition, the BG values referred to here are those using the American measurement standard of *mg/dL*, for milligrams per deciliter. The international standard is *mmol/L*, or millimoles/liter. Many glucose meters now allow you to switch between these two standards by pushing a button or setting a programming option. So hopefully you won't need to pull out your calculator to do the math yourself. But just in case you do, the conversion formulas are:

**To convert mg/dL of glucose to mmol/l, divide by 18
or multiply by 0.055.**

To convert mmol/L of glucose to mg/dL, multiply by 18.

Now, let's get started aiming you on the right path toward the long and healthy life you want.

PART

1

Getting a Handle on Your Health

1 You Have Diabetes:
What Now?!

"You Have Diabetes"—This Book Can Help

FINDING OUT THAT you or a loved one has diabetes can be pretty bad news, to be sure. Maybe you've been ignoring it or struggling with it for many years, and feeling pretty crummy. And all the negative headlines about diabetes and heart disease, kidney and nerve damage, blindness, etc., etc., certainly don't help. But here's the good news: for whatever it's worth, now is the best time ever to have diabetes. The "toolbox" of treatments is fuller than ever, and there are more programs, more classes, conferences, company resources, and a bigger support community available to you now than any time ever in history for any disease. But even with so many resources, most people don't feel upbeat about having diabetes. In fact, many hardly know where to start.

Knowing where you stand with your diabetes is the most important first step to outliving this disease. By outliving, we mean preventing the long-term complications of diabetes, and finding a way to manage your diabetes every day without going crazy, and without letting it rule your life. You will start by determining your results from five simple, common tests that will tell you your present risk for developing future problems:

- your hemoglobin A1c
- blood pressure
- lipids
- microalbumin
- eye exam

These will be introduced in detail in the following chapters. For each risk area that needs to be addressed, there are several approaches that have been shown to be effective. The great majority of people find that there are several important risk areas in which they are already doing quite well—areas that they need to know about, but about which they will not need to take immediate action. By focusing on your own one or two most significant health risks, you will more effectively improve your diabetes management, and avoid being overwhelmed by the notion that you have to tackle everything at once.

WHAT IS DIABETES?

DIABETES IS A disease in which the blood sugar, or **blood glucose (BG)**, is higher than normal, which can cause damage to various parts of the body over time.

Glucose is the common fuel used by all of your body's cells. **Insulin** is the hormone that controls the amount of glucose in your blood, and the amount that enters your cells to serve as fuel. Diabetes occurs when your body either does not make enough insulin (type 1), or because you become resistant to the effects of the insulin your body is producing (type 2).

See chapters 13 and 14 for details on type 2 and type 1 diabetes, respectively.

This book is designed to help people with type 2 diabetes successfully manage their own health—although anyone with diabetes can benefit from taking control of their five essential health factors.

Most people view diabetes as worse than it should be. This is because they are (1) worried about the serious complications that they hear about everywhere, and (2) overwhelmed by the difficult and numerous actions required of them. This view is understandable, as we are surrounded by news of the increasing impact of the diabetes "epidemic," and snowed under by the many unpleasant actions various experts propose we are supposed to take: lose weight, don't eat this, don't eat that, check your BG (when? seemingly all the time!), start going to the gym, and oh, have you lost thirty pounds yet? But this dreary approach actually points down the wrong road. Recent clinical studies confirm the value of a better, more accurate approach: Patients with diabetes do not need to do everything under the sun to live longer and healthier lives than ever before. They just need to learn the results of five tests, which point you in the right direction for protecting your future health.

Ten Things You Should Know about Diabetes

BEFORE WE GET started talking about how to treat it, let's talk a little about diabetes itself. How much do you really know about your disease? In your day-to-day life, you probably only think about the symptoms—mainly high BG levels—and how they make you feel, without having a firm grasp of the chemistry behind them. You probably also hear diabetes mentioned often in the media, discussed with varying levels of accuracy. Here are ten true things you should know about diabetes:

1. Diabetes is not itself a leading cause of blindness, but *poorly managed* diabetes is a leading cause of this and other serious health problems.
2. Thanks to an ever-wider range of effective approaches and treatments for diabetes, the long-range health complications such as heart disease, stroke, amputations, eye and kidney problems can be successfully avoided.

3. Diabetes is not your fault—type 2 diabetes is caused largely by a genetic propensity for insulin resistance and insulin deficiency.
4. Exercise (physical activity) has the single biggest positive effect on your diabetes.
5. Losing weight is not necessarily essential, but learning more about your food intake is essential.
6. You should eat a variety of foods, and there are no foods that are entirely off-limits.
7. Taking pills or insulin doesn't mean your diabetes is "worse"; your treatment doesn't tell you how severe your diabetes is—your test results do.
8. Insulin is actually a more natural treatment than any of the pills, and the injections don't hurt.
9. Patients with diabetes are living longer and healthier lives than ever, and all of the complications are decreasing in incidence.
10. Your doctor doesn't treat your diabetes—you do.

Sorting Facts from Myths

WITH THE LIST above in mind, be aware that much of what you have heard about diabetes is false, or does not apply to you and your diabetes.

Some things you might hear or believe, but they are, in fact, *baloney*:

- You can never eat sweets.
- You have to give up all the foods that taste good.
- Taking pills means that your diabetes is worse, and taking insulin: *yikes!*
- Complications will occur no matter what you do.
- Diabetes is insurmountable; even if you follow all the recommendations, diabetes will ruin your life in the end.

- Your poor lifestyle choices caused the diabetes; at least that's what your spouse says.

Two facts you don't often hear, but they are actually *happy truths*:

- With a little effort on your part, diabetes complications can be clearly avoided.
- The things you need to do to achieve good health may be easier than you think, and you have probably done some of them already.

A Step-by-Step, Positive Approach to Controlling Your Own Health

WHY ARE PATIENTS with diabetes are achieving longer, healthier lives than ever before? A decade or so ago, they were handed drug prescriptions and a strict generic meal plan, and sent home. Whoever who didn't follow doctor's orders to the letter was labeled "noncompliant." Moreover, they were expected to tackle all their health issues at once (diet, weight loss, BGs, blood pressure, etc.) and, even then, were given no assurance that they'd ever enjoy good health again.

We've come a long way, baby. Life is only getting better for people with diabetes, on many fronts, but you can successfully chart your own course for your specific diabetes. How? By becoming aware of the essential health numbers at your fingertips—a continuous health "report card" that you can improve upon in the various ways discussed in this book.

Our point is that you don't have to tackle everything at once. You can take it step-by-step. And in fact, there are some steps you personally may not need to take at all. Those that you do, you can custom-design to fit well into your lifestyle. Having diabetes does not mean you have to give up things you enjoy.

REAL PEOPLE:
DON'T SHUT DOWN BEFORE YOU GET STARTED

NED, A COMPUTER programmer in his mid-thirties with type 2 diabetes, was living the typical computer-nerd life: dining on pizza and regular Coke late in the evening, and often staying up all night to finish projects. Luckily for him, his boss also had diabetes and became concerned about his health.

The boss organized for the company to subsidize a visit to a weeklong diabetes education course. While this was good news for Ned, he became very nervous about participating in an immersion class in which he was sure he'd be put on a diet of rice cakes and vegetables, forced to exercise for hours, and generally have to give up all the treats he enjoyed. So in anticipation of this, Ned began indulging. In the one month before the program started, he gained an additional fifteen pounds.

When the class finally began, he was surprised to find that the first order of business was having his five risk factors tested. He learned that his A1c was a respectable 7.2, but his blood pressure and cholesterol levels were dangerously high.

Rather than recommending some birdseed diet, the course directors mainly advised him to change his fat intake, and start a moderate exercise routine, to bring down his blood pressure and cholesterol levels.

Ned was incredibly relieved: he did not have to change is life drastically after all. In fact, the changes he needed to make were pretty small and quite doable.

Keep an open mind about what you might need to do to improve your health. Don't give up before you get started.

You Can Find Your Own Individual Path

HERE ARE SOME things you will definitely need to do to get started (they're pretty simple):

- Spend a little time finding out more about your individual health risk factors that may be associated with future problems.
- Keep an open mind: be prepared to think about your activity and food in somewhat different ways than you do currently.
- Likewise, you may wish to try some new or different medications (always discuss this step with your health-care professionals before actually changing your drug regimen).
- Find a time and place to perform physical activity (this one's crucial).
- Understand that, with a little attention, especially soon after your diabetes diagnosis, you can benefit your health enormously.

As noted, the really good news is that there are some steps you personally may not need to take at all, or some that just come naturally as you follow your own path to improved health. For example, if your blood pressure or triglycerides are already under control, you can check off those items and move along to addressing a more pressing health issue. Note that your path is unique; it may be very different from what someone else diagnosed with diabetes needs to do. And your path will take some twists and turns over time, as your life situation and diabetes progression changes.

Learning to take care of your health is like learning to drive; with good driving skills, you can successfully navigate your own road, and even take your own detours if need be. Taking control of your diabetes is therefore not a one-time deal but an ongoing program. Still, just by knowing and taking action on some important basics, you can get a handle on your overall health faster and more successfully than you might think.

THE GOOD NEWS IN A NUTSHELL

> **THE BOTTOM LINE** is that, with the results of five essential tests and all the treatment choices available today, you can live well with diabetes in a way that no previous generation ever could.

Start by Setting Stress-Free Goals

WHAT ARE YOUR goals? Are you really committed to losing weight, or are you mainly interested in living a long and healthy life? Some experts assert that just telling someone to lose weight is a feeble approach from the doctor's side. Any diabetes doctor who's up to snuff should know that tremendous stress is associated with lifestyle changes, and sometimes just attempting to follow doctor's orders is not enough.

Be realistic: if changing your diet is too problematic, maybe you should work first on only increasing your exercise. But if you are a person who has a ten-hour workday or the primary caregiver for small children, you may not be able to dedicate the necessary time to an exercise program. Perhaps instead you can ask your doctor if you can try using an oral drug to lower your glucose levels. Or maybe you should focus on careful eating, and squeezing in a half-hour walk on your lunch break whenever possible. Goals have to be realistic for your *everyday* life. Trying to live up to a regimen that you find uncomfortable is counterproductive to accomplishing your goals. What's also important is this: You cannot just have any unhealthful lifestyle you want and assume that your medications will "take care of" the diabetes. You need to take at least some little actions to help your body's ability to optimally process those meds.

MEASURING YOUR SUCCESS

AS WE DISCUSS your goal-setting and strategies in this book, we'll refer to levels of success measured by these three factors:

RESULTS—the word we use to refer to your "numbers," or the immediate results of your laboratory tests and examinations (or results of clinical studies).

ACTIONS—defined as the physical things that you will do to improve your own health, such as exercising, eating different foods, and/or taking medications.

OUTCOMES—refers here to the consequences of your results and actions—in other words, the fact that you feel well, are becoming physically fit, and remain complication free.

Gaining Confidence Is Key: Use the CHECK Points

YOU'VE PROBABLY ALREADY done some things to effectively improve your health. If your blood pressure, weight, or cholesterol levels are in check, then you can be thankful to those areas don't need immediate attention. When addressing the areas where your test results do indicate health risks, be aware that little changes can make a big difference to the length and quality of your life.

If you've already made some changes and haven't seen improvement, this does not mean you have failed. Maybe you're focusing on something that is unrealistic for you. Or maybe it's time to introduce something new, like adding a drug that your doctor hasn't prescribed for you before, adding healthy snacks to your diet instead of eliminating all snacks and feeling deprived, asking a family member to help with time-consuming chores so that you can spend the free time exercising, or even working on stress reduction by trying meditation. Whatever it is, this new approach should change the way that you feel about your diabetes.

Sometimes lack of confidence is the biggest barrier to taking positive action. If you don't really believe that you can gain control of your own health, how can you stick to your goals? Well, we have an acronym for you. Even if you don't memorize the initial letters, the following five "CHECK Points" summarize this affirmative approach:

CONFIDENCE   You can make the lifestyle changes necessary to be successful.

HOPE   You can feel better now and in the future; you can live a long, healthy life with diabetes.

EFFICACY   You believe that the actions you take will be effective—that *your* actions, not just your doctor's, matter.

CLARITY   You can develop a plan for exactly what you need to do to succeed with diabetes.

KNOWLEDGE   You can gain an understanding of your diabetes that can serve and guide you.

Confidence—You may have thought that many diabetes-related lifestyle changes related to food, activity, weight, and checking your blood glucose would be just too difficult to accomplish. You will learn here that there are a number of different ways to reach the same goal, which is a long and healthy life. If you were driving your car toward some desired destination, and you ran into a roadblock, you wouldn't just sit there or try to drive through the roadblock. You would simply find another route around it. We want you to understand that there are different routes that will take you to your goal, and that at least some of them will be quite manageable.

Hope—Many individuals with diabetes feel doomed; they feel certain that complications are bound to happen. You may have relatives or friends with diabetes who've suffered debilitating complications and believe that your diabetes will end in the same manner. Or you may feel that the burden of diabetes is too much for you in your present life situation. Although these are common feelings, you do not have to dread a dark future. The fact is, everyone with diabetes can prevent some if not all complications. And it's not necessarily a question of just doing *more*, but rather a question of appropriately addressing your own biggest health issues, as outlined in this book. It is clear that patients with diabetes who make the effort to control their risk factors continue to improve their outcomes, and that this trend will be even more pronounced in the future as ever more is learned about this disease.

Efficacy—There is ample evidence that the approach described in this book will enable you to improve your own health. We know, for instance, that if your blood pressure is high, it can always be lowered into a safer range. You just need to find the right combination of lifestyle changes and medication that are effective for you at this point in time.

Clarity—It's important to know where to start, what changes to begin with, and how to measure whether you have achieved your target. This often means narrowing your focus, and beginning with one or two high-priority areas. It also means not spending energy on areas that are frustrating and nonessential. You may need to try a few approaches before you nail the one that works best for you. When you know how to actually get where you're going, you're more likely to get there.

Knowledge—Understanding the utility of the five diabetes-associated risk tests and what they tell you about your own diabetes, is the base on which to build your diabetes management plan. Understanding the different tools (activity, food, medications, and stress reduction) that affect each of these areas allows you to produce the plan best suited to you and your diabetes. There is more practical knowledge and research information about diabetes available than ever before. Two things the research tells us are: (1) type 2 diabetes is very heterogeneous (diverse among patients), and (2) it varies in even the same individual over time. This is why it doesn't make sense for everyone with diabetes to follow the same regimen, and why you will probably need to change your approach as time goes by. This book is designed to give you the knowledge you'll need to make beneficial adjustments in your diabetes care regimen throughout your long, happy life.

REAL PEOPLE:
LIFESTYLE CHANGES CAN MAKE YOU FEEL GOOD

JIM, A GENTLEMAN in his fifties, was extremely worried when he was diagnosed with type 2 diabetes. He had a family history of the disease, and his relatives had not fared well with it. Immediately, he felt defeated, dreading what lay ahead.

But he didn't want to give up altogether, so he went to see a specialist at a leading diabetes treatment center. He discussed exercise and diet with his doctor, and together they selected several achievable changes Jim could make to his regular routine.

On his next visit, one month later, Jim reported that he'd started walking and going to gym several times a week. He was using his monitor, and could see that his glucose levels had improved.

And here's the remarkable thing: Jim felt great. He explained that two things had changed his attitude: (1) he felt lucky to *know* that he had diabetes early on, so he had the impetus to work on improving his health—instead of waiting until he or his brother had a heart attack as a wake-up call, and (2) he realized that the lifestyle changes he needed to make for his diabetes were having an extremely positive effect on his overall well-being.

Rather than feeling like a punishment, eating more healthfully and exercising regularly can be a blessing in disguise, because you'll have increased energy and a better outlook on life.

2

What to Do First:
Discover Your Five Magic Numbers

Why and How to "Find Out Where You Are"

YOUR DIABETES DIAGNOSIS presented you with a load of things to worry about, both immediate and long term. The immediate concerns: having to monitor and change your diet and your level of physical activity, needing to check your blood glucose (BG), and wondering how to fit all of this work into your daily life. We will address these particular hurdles later in this book. For now, keep in mind what your diabetes regimen is for: these daily concerns will help you avert the serious long-term damage that poorly controlled diabetes can cause to your health.

In chapter 1, we talked about finding your own path to care for your health. Before you can discover that path, you need to find out where you are. In this case, we don't mean *where you are* in some spiritual sense, but in a much more precise way, based on our current scientific knowledge of diabetes risks.

You find your present "Diabetes Location" by learning the results of five specific tests, listed below. These five values will be your personal "Essential Health Factors"—or magic numbers—for living a long and healthy life with diabetes. That makes them pretty darn important.

The five tests are your:

- **Hemoglobin A1c**—a measure of the average amount of glucose in your blood over the last several months.
- **Blood Pressure**—a quick, painless armband test to determine the force of blood flow through your body.
- **Lipid Profile**—a group of blood tests measuring your cholesterol and triglycerides (another type of fat), which is used to determine your risk of heart attack or stroke.
- **Microalbumin**—a urine test that is an early indicator of kidney damage.
- **Eye Exam**—a yearly exam that consists of dilating your pupil, allowing the doctor to see the back of your eye.

The results of these tests will provide you with the baseline information you need. This chapter will walk you through understanding each test and show you how to create a personalized table of your results. We'll call this table "Your Diabetes Health Account," because it will clearly show you which areas are your health "assets" and which are your "debts" (or your biggest health risks). Although very simple, the table will track your most vital, life-saving information.

Keep in mind that you cannot evaluate your long-term risk of diabetes complications without first understanding your present status. Knowing where you stand now is the only way to determine the most useful next steps to take in order to achieve the long and healthy life you want. Just as you have your own unique goals in life, you'll have your own unique health profile revealed by these five tests. You'll be more in control, and probably feel more upbeat, the minute you start viewing your diabetes care from that perspective.

DON'T JUDGE YOUR HEALTH BY APPEARANCES

ONE DAY, TWO daughters from New Jersey brought their reluctant sixtyish mother, Marion, into a leading diabetes clinic. They were clearly quite concerned about the poor state of her diabetes care—convinced that her failure to eat right and exercise was slowly killing her.

Marion's husband, Karl, was also along, and had diabetes as well. But the daughters weren't concerned about him, because he was lean, and he exercised and ate well regularly. Yet when asked, Karl didn't have any idea of his latest A1c result.

Both parents underwent the five key risk factor tests. And guess what? Marion had an A1c of 7.6, which is not too shabby for someone supposedly slacking off. Karl, on the other hand, had an A1c of 8.4, which is relatively high, especially for someone who *thinks* he has optimal control.

As it turned out, Marion had to make a few changes, but Karl needed to take more actions to move his A1c out of the risk zone.

Clearly, appearances—or even actions such as exercising—are not enough to tell you where you stand with your diabetes. Without intervention, the husband in this story might have developed complications or even died before his wife. And everyone would have been shocked by Karl's unexpected demise.

It's not just about how you feel, or what others think.
Only your test results can tell you the true state of your health.

What We Know about Diabetes Complications

WHAT ARE THE future complications that you might face with type 2 diabetes? The one most likely to have a major impact is cardiovascular disease (the term *cardiovascular* combining heart disease and stroke). Remember that heart disease is also the leading cause of death in people without diabetes. But people with diabetes need to be especially careful, and can drastically reduce their risk by keeping their BG and blood pressure levels in check. The same is true for avoiding eye disease, kidney disease, nerve damage, and foot problems.

Although diabetes-related complications may seem to appear suddenly, they are actually the outcome of long periods—years and sometimes decades—of suboptimal metabolic control; that is, the total balance of the body's physical and chemical processes. What this means is that complications set in gradually, after the amounts of sugar, fats, and other substances in the blood have remained off balance for long periods of time.

One implication of this is that occasional high BG results are never directly worrisome; everyone has a few bad days now and then. However, if your levels *consistently* remain out of range, you are actively increasing your chance of future health problems.

So if your question is, "What are my chances of developing future complications from my diabetes?" the answer lies in the results of the five key tests we've just introduced. How can we be so sure? Just to be clear: this approach is not something we dreamed up on our own, but rather the clear-cut, commonly accepted results of multiple clinical studies.

Your Five Key Tests and What They Mean

Your A1c

What is the A1c?

The hemoglobin A1c is the single most important test for individuals with diabetes. It very accurately reflects your average BG values over the last three months. This average is measured as a percentage of the amount of sugar attached to your hemoglobin molecules, which are present in your red blood cells.

How does this work exactly? Think in terms of sticky sugar. In the body, sugar is also sticky, and clings particularly to proteins. The red blood cells that circulate in your body live for about three months before dying off. So the amount of sugar (glucose) stuck to these cells gives us an idea of how much sugar has been circulating in your blood for the past three months. The reason your A1c result is so important is that it's currently the only measure available that gives a view of your ongoing BG levels over the course of time—versus a single finger stick test with a home glucose meter, which only gives you a "snapshot" of your BG level at the very moment you test.

Note that this longer-term test was formerly called by a number of different names, including HbA1c, glycohemoglobin, glycated hemoglobin, and HbA1. Thankfully, the powers that be got together a few years ago and agreed to refer to it simply as the *A1c*.

Also, A1c laboratory results are more straightforward today than in the past, when there was a fair amount of confusion due to use of different measuring techniques. Today, the standardized range of A1c values for people *without* diabetes is 4.0 to 6.0 percent.

How and when is the test done?

The A1c is usually performed as a simple blood test, available at any medical laboratory or even onsite in some physicians' offices. Since the A1c reflects your glucose values over the last several months, there is no need to fast in preparation for the test, nor is it much affected by what you have eaten during the last several days, nor even by a recent history of high BG results.

You should have this test done at least every three months, and perhaps more often if you are making changes in your diabetes regimen and want to be able to gauge the effects of these changes. Although the A1c is affected by your BGs from the last several months, about half of the value reflects your BG average from just the last month. So if you have just initiated a new exercise program, made some healthy food changes, or added a new medication, you should be able to assess the impact by repeating your A1c test a little sooner than usual. (See chapter 5 for more details about the A1c test.)

What should your results be?

★ We generally recommend an A1c value of 7.0 percent or less. But your personal target may vary. This is one of the most important topics to discuss with your health-care provider. Everyone should know his or her individual A1c target (which may vary over time) as well as its most recent value.

■ Current recommendations from the American Diabetes Association (ADA) and the World Health Organization (WHO) are for a target of 7.0 percent for most diabetes patients. However, the American Association of Clinical Endocrinologists (AACE) is pushing for a more aggressive goal of 6.5 percent, though this lower target is not based on any new data. No clinical studies have shown that 6.5 or even 6.0 percent produces a significant health improvement over 7.0 percent, and it is unlikely that any clinical trial will be able to confirm a difference in this range.

What is the impact on your health?

Large-scale, long-term research studies show that lowering your A1c reduces your chance of all types of diabetes complications. This means that wherever your A1c may stand at the moment, any bit you can reduce it toward the target range makes you a much healthier person.

Study results actually showed that reducing your A1c from 9.0 to 7.0 cuts your chance of complications by about 70 percent. This positive effect continued for participants even after the study ended and their A1c values began to rise. In fact, in one major study, the protective effects of the lower A1c (averaging 7.1 in the treatment group), could still be seen ten years and longer after the study ended, even though the group's average A1c gradually increased to around 8.0. Conversely, we also know that when your

A1c remains high over long periods of time, your chance of complications increases significantly.

Still, despite the risk associated with higher A1c values, it is not absolutely certain that complications will occur. More and more people with diabetes are living longer and longer. Studies show that some diabetes patients who have survived for more than fifty years without major complications did not achieve ideal A1c results (as observed in the Joslin Diabetes Center's fifty-year insulin medalists study). The medical community's best guess on why this occurred is that these people have some genetic differences we don't yet understand. Somehow, some folks just get lucky. (It's even more remarkable that these patients achieved the results they did without the help of modern medications and know-how, including the A1c test, which has only been in common use for the last twenty-five years.)

But since we are unable to predict which individuals will be lucky enough to avoid complications, the idea is that all people with diabetes should work to optimize their A1c results. Remember that even small improvements in your A1c can help protect you from future problems.

THINK OF THE A1C AS YOUR SEATBELT LAW

LET'S EQUATE THE "low A1c rule" with the automobile seatbelt law—something everyone is required to do for protection. Some people will be lucky enough to avoid accidents, so the fact that they were foolish enough not to wear a seatbelt may not harm them. But that's largely up to chance. No one can predict whose luck might turn for the worse, for whom a possible complication may throw a curve in the road. By keeping your A1c in range, you can *ensure* a healthy future. As they say, "An ounce of protection is worth a pound of cure."

Note that while checking your BG day-to-day remains an essential step in your daily diabetes care, your A1c result always provides more accurate and more important information about your ongo-ing, long-term BG control. Whenever the question is, "Are my BG results increasing or decreasing my chances of future complica-tions?" the answer is, "What is my A1c?"

Your Blood Pressure

What is high blood pressure?

Be aware of your blood pressure. That is one of the most impor-tant messages in this book. Blood pressure is an underappreciated diabetes risk factor. Most people realize that it is somehow impor-tant to their health, but often neither they nor their health-care providers recognize its fundamental role in predicting cardiovas-cular risk, particularly for people with diabetes. Blood pressure is reported as two numbers, such as 120/80. The top number is called the *systolic*, and the bottom number the *diastolic*. Both numbers are important in assessing cardiovascular risk.

As you might imagine, blood pressure that is too high puts extra stress on your arteries. (The blood vessels that carry blood directly from your heart to your body's organs are the *arteries*; the blood vessels that return your blood to your heart are your veins.) Over time, this extra stress on the arteries leads to higher risk of heart attack or stroke.

A study performed in Great Britain over a period of more than ten years illustrated this very clearly. The study examined dia-betes-related complications in almost four thousand patients with type 2 diabetes. The results again confirmed the positive effect of lowering A1c values on reducing complications but, in addition, they showed that lowering blood pressure had an even greater effect on decreasing diabetes-related complications.

For every 10-point drop in the systolic blood pressure (the top number), there was almost a 20 percent decrease in the chance of stroke, and a 15 percent decrease in the chance of heart attack. This benefit did not bottom out at the current national target of

130; there was continued benefit to lowering the blood pressure to 120 and further.

Knowing your blood pressure, and getting it into your target range is extremely effective and important for your health. Fortunately, there are an increasing number of medications available to help reduce blood pressure, if needed. Nowadays we also better understand the impact of exercise and food on blood pressure.

How and when is the test done?

This test is conducted routinely in doctor's offices, probably every time you visit the doctor for any kind of checkup. The test is very simple and comfortable. A cuff is wrapped around your upper arm, and slowly inflated. The cuff squeezes your arm more and more tightly until the pressure of the cuff is higher than the highest pressure in your artery, and the artery collapses under the pressure and stays closed. This may sound rough, but it doesn't hurt a bit.

The pressure in the cuff is then slowly decreased. The point at which the artery is able to pop open momentarily is what is called the systolic pressure (the highest pressure reached by the pumping heart). As the pressure in the cuff decreases further, it reaches a point at which the artery is able to remain continuously open. This point is the diastolic pressure, which is the lowest blood pressure reached when the heart is relaxing, and readying itself for its next contraction.

What should your results be?

★ We generally recommend a blood pressure value of 130/80 or lower, in accordance with the current recommendation of the American Diabetes Association and other national organizations.

■ However, available evidence shows that lower values are even more protective against cardiovascular risk. We think you can safely consider a goal of 125, or even 120 if you have other cardiovascular risk factors—including previous personal history of cardiovascular disease, family history of heart disease, smoking, high LDL or low HDL cholesterol, high triglycerides, and/or elevated microalbumin (see the sections that follow for explanations of these).

Your Lipids

What are lipids?

Most people have heard of cholesterol, but the term *lipids* may be less familiar. This term is commonly used to describe a group of three tests: LDL cholesterol, HDL cholesterol, and triglycerides. Each of these is a type of fat that circulates in your blood, and they have been linked—both individually and as a group—to increased risk of heart disease and stroke. Details of these tests are covered in chapter 5, where you will learn more about their practical significance.

Cholesterol was one of the first important risk factors identified for heart disease. Years ago, doctors could only take a measurement of "total cholesterol," which was rather imprecise. Nowadays, cholesterol is gauged using these three more precise measures: LDL (low-density lipoprotein) or "bad" cholesterol that tends to collect and build a thick, hard deposit that clogs your arteries; HDL (high-density lipoprotein) or "good" cholesterol that tends to carry cholesterol away from the arteries and back to the liver, thus slowing the buildup; and triglycerides, a creamy form of fat that comes from food and is also made in your body, which contributes to your total cholesterol results.

How and when is the test done?

This is another simple blood test, generally performed along with your A1c, as your doctor usually writes a combined lab order. In other words, one blood sample is sufficient for the lab to measure your LDL, HDL, and triglycerides. If you have concerns about your triglycerides, the test should be done following overnight fasting. LDL and HDL cholesterol are not much affected by food, however, so you don't need to be fasting if you're taking the test especially to monitor these lipids. Nevertheless, it is always bad form to show up for your blood test gripping a fast-food take-out sack, even if there was a two-for-one special. Don't laugh, as we've seen this happen! And the smell of french fries can be disconcerting in the lab.

What should your results be?

★ For people with type 2 diabetes, we recommend:
  - an LDL cholesterol target of 80 mg/dL or less
  - an HDL cholesterol target of 45 or more
  - a triglyceride target of under 150

■ Current American Diabetes Association guidelines recommend that LDL cholesterol be below 100. But since LDL is the most important risk factor of the three, and there is accumulating evidence that lower cutoffs are even more beneficial, we side with the National Cholesterol Education Program (NCEP) in recommending a more aggressive goal of 80.

HDL cholesterol targets are slightly different, because this element is associated with a *decreased* risk of cardiovascular disease. So you want a higher number for "good cholesterol." Some national groups recommend goals of over 40 for men and over 50 for women. But the evidence for gender distinction in goals for patients with diabetes isn't strong. In the general population, women are at lower risk for heart disease than men—yet women who have diabetes have the same cardiovascular risk as that of men. This is why we recommend a midpoint target that everyone can aim for: 45 or more.

Triglycerides differ from LDL and HDL cholesterol in that triglyceride levels increase following a meal, and stay elevated for several hours or more afterward. So triglycerides are usually tested after overnight fasting (generally after ingesting nothing but water for at least ten hours before the test, which should be conducted in the morning before 10 AM). If your triglyceride level isn't tested following fasting, but is still below 150, you are in good shape, because your fasting results would be even lower. If, however, your triglyceride level tested when you weren't fasting is above 150, you should have it rechecked when you are fasting. It will be lower and may then prove to be out of the danger zone.

Your Microalbumin

What is microalbumin?

This test searches for small amounts of a protein called *albumin*, which leaks into the urine when the kidneys are becoming damaged. Surprisingly, it is the test most frequently neglected in patients with diabetes, but is by far the most sensitive test for identifying risk of future kidney problems. It is also the most recent test to become available, appearing in the last fifteen years.

Until the advent of this test, the two tests available (urine protein and serum creatinine, the latter being a blood test) could only identify advanced-stage kidney damage. So by the time patients realized their test results were off target, they were already likely to develop end-stage kidney disease within the next five years. Bad news for patients.

The ultrasensitive microalbumin test is the earliest available indicator for the development of kidney disease, showing changes ten to twenty years earlier than older tests could. More importantly, numerous clinical studies show that when increases in microalbumin are identified early, a number of different treatments can be used to decrease or even eliminate your chance of developing kidney disease. These treatments include aggressive control of blood pressure, improvement in BG control, and using specific medicine classes such as ACE inhibitors and ARBs (see chapter 11 for a description of these drugs). Happily, these treatments have been responsible for the sharp decrease in incidence of kidney disease in patients with diabetes.

What should your results be?

★   We generally recommend a microalbumin result of 30 or less.

■   Note that the microalbumin test has not yet been standard-ized the way the A1c has, so results may vary by laboratory. The upper limit of the normal range hovers around 30, but the lower range can show quite a bit of variability. In fact, whether you are at 15, or even 5, on the low end doesn't make too much difference, and it doesn't matter much if your year-to-year results bounce around a bit, as long as you remain in the normal range. Even results that are minimally elevated may not be reproducible, so if you get a high reading, your first step might be to simply repeat the test for a double-check.

In addition, microalbumin tests that correct for the amount of creatinine in your urine are more accurate and reproducible. You should ask if this choice is available from your lab, and request it.

How and when is the test done?

This test is done using a urine sample, rather than blood. But it cannot be checked using the routine "dipstick" test offered in most medical offices. Although these dipsticks can measure pro-tein in the blood, they look only at the larger proteins, and are not very sensitive. You should have a test that specifically measures microalbumin, conducted in a laboratory setting.

In the past, and still sometimes in the present, your health-care provider may ask you to collect your urine for 24 hours for this test. This is not only cumbersome (actually, it's *really, really* cumber-some) but also unnecessary. Studies have shown that a random sin-gle urine sample is just as accurate, especially when the urine sample is also used to measure creatinine, so that the lab can report a microalbumin/creatinine ratio. If you want to learn more fasci-nating facts about collecting urine, please see chapter 5.

Your Eye Exam

What should your eye exam cover?

People with diabetes are frightened of losing their sight, for obvious reasons. We constantly hear that diabetes is the leading cause of blindness in adults, and none of us can imagine a life without vision. However, it is a slight misstatement to say that diabetes is the leading cause of blindness in adults; it would be more accurate to say that *poorly treated* diabetes is the leading cause. Again, studies clearly show that with regular screenings (once a year) by an eye doctor experienced in diabetes, eye changes can be detected very early and problems can be successfully treated and even reversed.

In fact, the major problem with preventing eye disease in people with diabetes is that most patients are not screened regularly; even people who wear glasses may have only their distance vision and ability to focus tested while being fitted, rather than having their eyes thoroughly examined for any physical deterioration. A second problem is that there is a lack of well-trained eye doctors to do a medical screening. While this is a general public health problem in the United States, you don't want to become a statistic of this problem. Insist on a full eye exam yearly, by an eye doctor experienced in detecting the early-stage changes that diabetes commonly causes in the back of your eyes, on the retinas, which is called *retinopathy*.

Left alone, this damage progresses from background retinopathy to **nonproliferative retinopathy**, and then to **preproliferative retinopathy**, which is the stage at which interventions with laser therapy are effective. But long before that, control of blood pressure and A1c are effective in halting the development of retinopathy—and can even help reverse early changes that may have already occurred.

As with each of the other four tests detailed above, the key is regular screenings. The early detection of eye problems allows you to achieve the maximum benefit from the many highly effective treatments available today.

How and when is the test done?

An eye exam should be performed annually by an experienced eye doctor, usually an ophthalmologist, and involves dilating the eye. *Dilation* means expanding the pupil of the eye so the doctor can see into the back area, where your sensitive retina is located. This is achieved using special eye drops that open up your pupil. You may need to wear dark glasses for a few hours after the exam, because until the drops wear off, your pupil won't be able to contract to protect your eyes from bright light.

If it turns out that the exam reveals you have signs of any eye problems associated with diabetes, you may need to see a retinal specialist, called a retinologist, for a more precise diagnosis and optimal treatment.

VIEW OF EYE AT ANNUAL EXAM

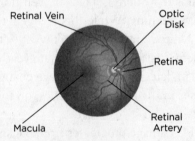

What should your results be?

★ The ideal result you are looking for here is: no evidence of retinopathy.

■ In contrast to the other tests, there is no numerical result from an eye exam, no "magic number" with an accompanying normal range. Instead, there are different grades of retinopathy, ranging from none to "background" to "nonproliferative" to "preproliferative," and further stages. Furthermore, most ophthalmologists don't provide you with detailed information about your exam results. Sometimes your eyes may show nonproliferative retinopathy, and yet you will be told that your eyes are okay.

What the ophthalmologist means in such a case is that there were no changes requiring immediate treatment, so why bother with labels or details? But to you, a change in status from no retinopathy to nonproliferative retinopathy is a significant one—a signal to take a close look at your other diabetes complication risk factors, and probably review your overall diabetes regimen. This is why it is vital that you consult an ophthalmologist who has experience with patients who have diabetes.

Even so, since there is no generally accepted system for reporting eye exam results to patients, even those with diabetes (a deficit that won't likely be corrected any time soon), you will probably have to do a little more work on your own to obtain your results from the doctor and interpret them. Feel free to insist that your eye doctor provide and explain any and all findings. For the most common diabetes-related eye problem, retinopathy, your eye doctor should be able to tell you with accuracy that you fall in one of several categories:

- No evidence of diabetic retinopathy
- Mild background diabetic retinopathy
- Nonproliferative diabetic retinopathy
- Preproliferative diabetic retinopathy
- Proliferative diabetic retinopathy

There are several subdivisions of each category here, but these are the main classifications. The last two may signal a need for laser therapy to the back of the eye, called *photocoagulation*. This therapy, when properly done, is very successful at slowing, stopping, and sometimes reversing retinopathy.

There are several other eye disorders that an ophthalmologist may discover, the most worrisome of which is **macular edema**. This is a buildup of fluid behind the *macula*, which is the portion of the retina most important for our vision, as it is the area that helps focus the images at which we are looking directly. Treatment here can be difficult, as this is the most sensitive part of the retina.

The other most common findings during an eye exam are signs of **cataracts**, a clouding of the eye lens or its surrounding transparent membrane, which obstructs the passage of light; or signs of **glaucoma**, which shows up as an enlarged "cup-disk ratio" caused by increased pressure from the fluid inside the eye. If either of these is suspected, further tests will be required to determine whether you need treatment. Not to worry. Both cataracts and glaucoma can be treated very successfully when diagnosed early.

REMEMBER:

- You can't get very specific help if you have no idea where your diabetes stands.
- You can't improve or maintain your health if you have no information about what your real risks are.

Get Your Test Results:
Create Your Personal Diabetes Health Account

WITH THE INFORMATION in this chapter as your guide, you are now ready to take the first steps toward finding out where you stand with your diabetes. The idea is to chart your test results, just as carefully as you track your personal wealth. We will help you create a simple balance sheet to see clearly where you have the most "health dollars in the bank" and where your most urgent debts lie. Remember, the more dollars you have, the more likely you are to live a long and healthy life with diabetes. It's your job to collect those dollars. And how do you get them? By knowing your test result numbers, and taking the most affective actions to improve them where needed.

First, do you have access to your current test results? It's very likely that you've had most of these tests done at some point, but less likely that you know what your results were, or exactly what they meant. Right? Here's a guide to recommended testing frequency, so you'll know if the numbers you have are current:

- the A1c blood test—*every three months*
- blood pressure—*every six months at least* (take advantage of every doctor's appointment to have this checked, especially if it's been elevated or you've had concerns)
- microalbumin, lipids, and eye exam—*all annually* (unless concerns call for more frequent checks)

If you've had these tests done within the last year (or the last four months at least for the A1c) and you have the results at hand, make a quick list of them.

If you don't have a written copy of your results for some or all of these tests, your first step is to retrieve them from your health-care provider. It is your right to request them, so don't feel intimidated about speaking up. A call to the office should suffice, although this seemingly simple task can sometimes be time-consuming and frustrating. Our recommendation is to make the call at a time when you have some other paperwork to do, and use a speakerphone, so that you don't get too frustrated trying to get through or waiting on the line (sound familiar?). The assistant should be able to look up at least one result—your blood pressure—from the office records, without taking the time to contact a lab.

Don't mess around with approximations. You need to know your *exact* results. For example, you almost certainly had your blood pressure measured at your last doctor's visit, but perhaps they only told you that your blood pressure was "okay" or "Not to worry, it's just high because you're nervous at the doctor's office." Perhaps they said that your blood pressure was 130/80. This was probably your approximate blood pressure, because the chance that both systolic and diastolic numbers end evenly in 0 is one in a hundred. Perhaps they measured a little too quickly, and what you really have is an estimate.

Or if you are told that your A1c is "good," that's nice, but not nearly precise enough. You wouldn't go to the bank asking for your account balance, and accept an answer that it was "pretty good." This is an important number that you need to know precisely.

Ideally, the results of every test should reach you in the form of the actual lab report, as a fax or an e-mail attachment, or even a photocopy sent to you in the mail, so that you can read for yourself everything detailed there. If you have questions, do not hesitate to ask your doctor to explain what the terms and numbers mean.

YOU ARE THE ONE WITH THE DIABETES

> **THESE NUMBERS BELONG to you, and knowing them is your right, as well as critical to your health—just like the numbers in your bank account.**

No cheating as you fill in your personal chart with the results. Even if you think a test result is higher than you'd like, and you want to change it, you need to know the real number. This chart is for you and your health only, so don't be ashamed to mark down whatever the numbers are, even if they're nothing near the ideal values. There's actually a good chance that your result is better than you think, and even if it isn't, you need to know your true starting point in order to begin making changes. Perhaps you've hit a bad period in your life, full of stresses and temporary setbacks. Still, you need to find out where you are—even if your plan is to just wait until you straighten out your job situation before you can get back to some of your health concerns.

You may find that some tests have not been done at all, particularly the microalbumin. Ask your doctor's office to schedule these tests for you. You won't need an office visit. They will be able to notify the lab, and you can just go directly there. For the lipid test, it is useful to go when you are fasting, which means the test should be done in the early morning before 10 AM, after you have gone at least ten hours without eating. (Pure water is okay, but coffee, tea,

YOUR DIABETES HEALTH ACCOUNT

	A1c Target	Your A1c	Blood (BP) pressure Target	Your BP	LDL	Your LDL	HDL	Your HDL	Triglycerides	Your Trigl	Microalbumin (MA)	Your (MA)	Eye Exam	Your Eye exam
(5 money bags)	≤ 6.5		≤ 120		≤ 80		≥ 55		≤ 80		≤ 30		No evidence of retinopathy	
(4 money bags)	≤ 7.0		≤ 130		≤ 100		≥ 45		≤ 150		≤ 30		Minimal of retinopathy	
(3 money bags)	≤ 8.0		≤ 135		≤ 120		< 45		≤ 250		≤ 40		Minimal of moderate	
(1 money bag)	≤ 9.0		≤ 140		≤ 140				200-400		40-300		Pre-proliferative	
PAST DUE	> 9.0		> 140		> 140				> 400		> 300		Proliferative or macular edema	

soda, juice, and flavored waters are not.) Ask the lab personnel to send you your own copy of the results. They should be able to do so, but many labs are still stuck in Old World Medicine mode and will give you trouble. Legally, the results are yours, so give it a try at least; otherwise, work with your primary care physician's staff to secure a copy (the lab will have sent your results there).

For any tests conducted on-site in your doctor's office, you can insist on getting a photocopy right then and there, to take home with you when you leave. Once you have these results, place them into the chart provided here. At this point, the most important factor is not so much what your numbers are, but just the fact that you now know them.

Once you have filled out this chart, step back, and pat yourself on the back. You have several reasons to be proud. You have just made the first step toward living a long and healthy life with diabetes. This is true no matter what your results—because the amazing fact is that most people with diabetes do not know what their numbers are, or what they mean. So, congratulations. Whatever your numbers are, you can feel good about the initial accomplishment of knowing them.

Would you believe that a recent U.S. Department of Agriculture (USDA) outreach survey showed that, of more than seven thousand patients with type 2 diabetes, *fewer than 10 percent* had even a general idea of their last A1c result, and what it meant? The numbers for the microalbumin test were even lower. So, just by knowing your numbers and understanding what they mean, you're already at the head of the diabetes class—and the next steps you'll take will help you stay there.

Now Review Your Personal Balance Sheet

Take a look at your table. Where do you have the most "assets"? Most likely, there are one or more areas where you are pretty comfortable. Now comes the important part: in which areas are you running low, or even in debt? Debt signifies a serious health risk that you'll want to address immediately.

If you don't have a single debt area, take a deep breath and relax. You may have some work to do, but you are getting close to all-around success in your diabetes care. At the very least, you can take your time learning more about your diabetes, and what you may need to do in the future to maintain your good results.

If you do have some areas of debt, or some without a lot of savings, take heart: this is not a sign of failure. Rather, you are now aware of the red-flag areas where you need to make an investment in your health immediately. If you delay, the debt collector will soon come after you, in the form of damage to your nerves or eyes. So think about making these past-due areas your most immediate concern.

REAL PEOPLE:
YOUR TEST RESULTS
WILL DETERMINE YOUR ACTIONS

A WOMAN BROUGHT her two diabetic parents, Louise and Bill, into a big-city diabetes clinic from their farm in the Midwest. She was worried because, despite their diagnosis, her parents just couldn't seem to change their lifestyle. Both in their late sixties, they still ate greasy bacon and eggs for breakfast, and were now less physically active on the farm as they used to be. Tests revealed that both Louise and Bill's LDL levels were quite healthy, and both had an A1c under 7.0, which is quite good indeed. But they both had very high blood pressure—which neither parent nor their daughter had even considered for a moment in the past.

In response, the doctors recommended not changes in diet or exercise, but rather a more strict commitment to taking their blood pressure medications more regularly, and possibly adding other pills to the mix (to be determined by a specialist).

All three of them left the clinic feeling relieved and also astonished—because, without the testing, they would never have

> had the slightest idea that both Louise and Bill's most urgent
> health risk was high blood pressure.
>
> Without knowing your test results, you can only guess at what
> would be the right actions to improve your health.

Pinpoint Your Focus

Knowing your own diabetes state—what looks good, what needs urgent attention, and what needs some work over time—will enable you to pinpoint the focus of your actions. This means the end of vague resolutions like "I'll eat better" or "I'll lose ten pounds soon." Instead, you can focus on very specific improvements like lowering your A1c by checking your BG more often so that you can react immediately to highs—or getting your systolic blood pressure down from 150 to 140.

The next chapter will lead you through developing a personalized plan of action. We'll recommend specific steps you can take to improve your health in the areas where you need it most. Often, you will have a choice of actions. And most important, you will be able to monitor your success just by keeping track of your five key values.

You don't have to start right this minute, but probably sometime this week. It might be as simple as scheduling an eye exam, talking to your health-care provider about medications, or figuring out some practical lifestyle changes you can make right way.

DON'T THINK YOU HAVE TO TACKLE EVERYTHING AT ONCE

> THE RISK TABLE is designed to help you and your doctor pin-
> point which *one or two* things you need to focus on improving
> in the coming months.

3

What to Do Next:
Plan for Action

Prioritize Your Health Debts

NOW THAT YOU are armed with the knowledge of where your diabetes stands, you can start making real, substantial improvements right away.

First, look over Your Diabetes Health Account from chapter 2. Remember, if some of your results are missing, or the tests haven't been done recently, call right now to schedule them. Even if the tests can't be done soon, having the appointments in place ensures that you are making headway in improving your health wealth, so to speak. And there are certainly some areas where you already have money in the bank:

- If you have four to five moneybags: Good work. This means these items aren't posing any health risk for you at the moment. Just keep an eye on your "account balance" over time to make sure it remains high.
- If you have one or two moneybags only: these are action items, indicating areas of concern, and should be addressed as soon as you've "paid off your debts."

- If any debts are "past due": Urgent! These items need your immediate attention.

Rather than depressing you, knowing your priorities should boost your confidence; you have learned *exactly* which health factors are most important for you right now, and which may not need attention on an everyday basis.

Now comes the interesting part: based on your numbers, it's time to choose *one or two* high-priority actions that you *are* going to focus on initially in order to make improvements. You'll need to be very specific about exactly what you'll do and when, steps you'll need to take, and how these new actions will fit into your daily life.

Strategies for Improvement That You Can Cycle Through

WE'RE GOING TO give you some advice that's hard to come by: how you can get the "biggest bang for your buck" when improving your health. We're going to begin by laying out the key improvement strategies for each health marker (or risk area), in a step-by-step process starting with the lifestyle changes you can easily make, and then cycle through to more aggressive ways that will bring your results into the target range. If the first recommendation doesn't yield results for you, you can move on to the second, and so on.

As you read, you'll notice that most of these treatment strategies are related to each other; for example, the exercise and food changes you make for lowering your A1c will improve all four of your other health factors as well.

What Can You Do to Improve Your A1c?

1. **You might be surprised to learn that the most effective tool for glucose control is activity—any type of activity that moves your body through space.** The most common form of exercise is walking, which can be done outdoors, inside at a shopping

mall, or on a treadmill, as long as your legs are moving you forward. The amount of walking required to benefit your diabetes may be less than you think. Frequency is also important: doing some kind of regular movement at least four times a week may be crucial, if you are otherwise fairly inactive. Note that intermittent activity also works well; ten minutes of exercise twice a day has a similar effect on your diabetes as twenty minutes once a day. Exercise has an immediate effect on lowering your BG, and also has the beneficial long-term effect of reducing your insulin resistance. If you're able to exercise four times a week or more, the effects of that activity will last you the whole week long. (See chapter 7 for more on the power of exercise.)

2. **Which foods to eat, of course, is a major concern for everyone living with diabetes.** We know that the most important factor is the type of food you eat, and the good news is that a wide variety fits well with diabetes. You need to learn a little about how different foods affect your BG, as this will go a long way toward keeping your A1c in check. For glucose control, understanding carbohydrates is crucial. Carbohydrates are foods either made up primarily of sugar or those that convert to sugar in your system, such as starches like potatoes and pasta. Knowing the types and amounts of carbohydrates in your food is a critical step to deciding what changes, if any, to make in your food choices.

3. **Next most important is portion size, which is difficult these days when everything is supersized.** There are lots of books to help you learn to measure and/or eyeball your portions in order to keep from overeating. And do you really know what a "balanced meal" is? It's a mix of carbohydrates, protein sources, and fibrous foods like beans and vegetables—ideally not too much of anything at one sitting. Learn more about diabetes and food in chapter 8.

4. **Stress is another major factor: both the stress related to your diabetes, and other stresses in your life that might be making it**

harder to focus on your glucose control. Exercise is an excellent stress-buster, plus you can try anything that suits you: enjoying inspirational books, movies, and music; seeing a counselor; or practicing stress reduction through meditation. In this arena, too, there are more options available to help you than ever before.

5. **Finally, you can and will probably move up the ladder of medication options as time goes by.** Diabetes itself changes in a person's body over time: insulin production by your pancreas decreases, and insulin resistance may also increase. This is important to keep in mind, because an increase in your A1c may well be related to a change in your underlying diabetes, rather than to anything you did wrong. When this occurs, there are a number of safe, well-studied medications that work on the underlying disease process to improve your glucose control. As you will learn in chapter 9, there are five main classes of medications for type 2 diabetes, including three major types of oral medications, incretins in different forms, plus insulin, which is also available in several forms, the newest being inhalable. As your diabetes progresses over time, you will likely need to cycle through these choices, gradually adding new medications, and also changing the dosages of current medications. Although the great number of new, effective medications has had the biggest impact in improving glucose results among patients in general—it is your continuing attention to activity and food that provides the foundation for their effectiveness. The medications are great helpers, but you will still have to do some work as outlined above, to stay healthy.

If you are in debt, with an A1c over 9.0

An A1c over 9.0 is generally considered a significant health debt. This is because your chance of diabetes-related complications is over three times higher than it would be if your A1c were at 7.0.

The good news here is that getting your A1c down to 8.0 or lower is a fairly straightforward affair. Your first step is to honestly assess your present lifestyle and medications, and discuss this immediately with your doctor or diabetes educator.

If you have an A1c of 9.0 or above, your doctor will probably suggest additional glucose-lowering medications. You may already have some of these, but perhaps you've stopped taking them, or are not taking them regularly. If you are taking your current prescriptions properly, then your doctor may need to step up your drug regimen by prescribing higher dosages or new medications.

The next most vital consideration here is your current level of physical activity. When you first begin exercising, there may be a lag period before it shows its full effect. But make no mistake: exercise is an essential component to your diabetes management.

Finally, you may need to turn a practical eye to your present food intake. Has the volume of your eating changed recently? And what changes can you make to your food choices? Be practical and start with small, incremental changes that you feel comfortable with, as big or unpalatable changes in your food patterns are harder to maintain over time.

In summary, your most important options for lowering your A1c are (1) increases in physical activity, and (2) changes in medication. Improving your food portions and food choices may also help.

REAL PEOPLE:
TAKING INSULIN CAN BE BETTER, NOT WORSE

> BRENDA, A SECRETARY in her mid-forties, had diabetes for six years and was moderately overweight. She signed herself up for a three-day diabetes management program at a local clinic, mainly because her A1c was steady at around 8.1 and her doctor kept saying she should start taking insulin, which she most certainly did not want to do.

The doctors and educators at the program also thought insulin would be a good choice for Brenda, but they saw her discomfort, and embraced it. Rather than lecturing her, they spent most of their time just talking with her, abating her common fears: that insulin means her diabetes is "worse," that the injections will hurt, that she'll suffer dangerous low blood sugars, that insulin is only for patients "nearing the end."

Finally, the team suggested that trying one injection would not mean Brenda was signed up for life; she could stop the insulin if it was unbearable for her. So they showed her how to draw from a vial using a syringe, and helped her take a shot of saline for practice at the clinic. Then they gave her real insulin supplies to take home and try.

The next day, Brenda returned to the program elated: she had managed to give herself a shot at home. And it didn't really hurt. And afterward, her blood glucose dropped to under 200 for the first time in ages.

Brenda was so relieved. In fact, her only regret was that she'd put off going on insulin for so long—because now she could see that it would provide better diabetes control and also make her feel much better, both physically and mentally.

Insulin is just another tool for improved diabetes care—one of the most effective, in fact. It can actually improve your quality of life along with your diabetes control.

What Can You Do to Improve Your Blood Pressure?

Note that people with type 2 diabetes are prone to high blood pressure, because insulin resistance tends to be coupled with high blood pressure and also makes it a little more resistant to treatment. For these reasons, it may sometimes be necessary to use multiple treatments to bring your blood pressure into the target range. On the positive side, research studies have shown that once you achieve your blood pressure target, by whatever means, you receive the same protective benefit as do people without diabetes. If your blood pressure is high, it may be more important to bring this under control than even your BG. For every 10 points that you reduce your systolic pressure (the top number), you will reduce your chance of heart attacks and strokes by 15 to 20 percent. This is an area where you can really put away some savings in your health account:

1. **Learn to check your blood pressure at home.** One of the most useful ways to improve your blood pressure is to know more about it. Whenever you have your blood pressure checked, ask for the result, and note it down if it is above your target range. If your blood pressure remains high despite some initial treatments, such as lifestyle changes or medications, you should begin to monitor it more closely yourself by purchasing a home monitoring kit. This will allow you to better follow the effect of further treatments you'll be trying. Home monitors are becoming much more reliable than in the past, and are available at most pharmacies and in the pharmacy sections of many large retail stores.

2. **A number of new medications have been introduced in recent years to treat high blood pressure.** Most have few side effects, meaning you have an array of choices to help you find an effect treatment. Some of these medications also have helpful secondary effects. For example, ACE inhibitors and ARBs protect the kidneys from damage, and beta blockers can decrease the chance of further heart problems in patients with a history of heart disease. See chapter 11 for an explanation of these drugs.

3. **Aerobic exercise has an additional benefit (beyond improving your glucose control) in reducing your blood pressure, when conducted regularly.** Although starting with any activity is useful, you will achieve the best effects when you are active

at least four days a week, with sessions of at least thirty minutes each day.

4. **Fruits and vegetables are more than just plain old healthy.** They are actually key dietary components to controlling your blood pressure. Several large clinical studies have shown that increasing the amount of fruits and vegetables in your diet—eating five or more servings per day—significantly decreases high blood pressure.

5. **Lowering your salt intake is also very helpful. You can decrease your intake not only by avoiding use of the salt shaker, but also by avoiding prepared foods with a high sodium content.** (Low sodium is defined as 140 mg per serving or less.) If a product contains 50 percent or more of your recommended daily total for sodium, try to find a lower-sodium substitute for it. Make sure to read those nutrition labels. (See chapter 8 for a how-to guide).

6. **Reducing stress by a variety of techniques also helps to lower blood pressure.** You can try relaxation activities such as meditation or yoga, if these appeal to you. Or sometimes simple choices—such as changes in your work or home environment—can make a difference. Maybe you can work with your boss to take some responsibilities "off your plate," or move your workspace at home into another area to cut down on the noise factor and distractions. It's worth thinking about the little things that aggravate you on a regular basis.

7. **Stop smoking.** Smoking has a direct effect on blood pressure, as well as direct harmful effects on your heart and brain—not to mention those non-diabetes-related issues such as lung cancer and emphysema. Smoking doesn't just make your blood pressure higher, it *doubles* your chance of developing heart disease and multiplies your chances of having a heart attack or stroke by *two to four times*. One of the most promising trends in diabetes treatment is that in recent years, patients with diabetes have cut down on smoking more significantly than the decrease in the general population. We

consider this an affirmation of (first doctor in the United States to successfully specialize in diabetes care) Dr. Elliott Joslin's early assertion that "people with diabetes tended to be smarter than the general population."

If you are in debt, with a systolic reading over 140

Systolic blood pressure over 140 is bad news. This increases your chance of heart disease and stroke, affects circulation in your legs, and contributes to eye and kidney disease. In most cases, you should start immediately on a blood pressure–lowering medication, even if you are already taking other medications. We know that many people prefer to work with lifestyle changes first. This approach is correct in general, but when your blood pressure is this high, you should not wait for the effects of your lifestyle changes to kick in. You can always reduce or stop the medication in the future if you are able to reduce your blood pressure even further through exercise, food changes, and/or stress reduction.

What Can You Do to Improve Your Lipids?

Lifestyle changes are always the first approach, mostly because they are very effective and the side effects are always beneficial. In fact, you may have noticed a pattern by now: the perks of starting exercise and improving your food choices—lowering insulin resistance, directly decreasing heart disease, decreasing depression, helping weight loss, improving arthritis, and so on—are excellent for combating all of your risk factors. So, try to:

1. **Change the types and amounts of fat in your diet.** Good fats can improve your cholesterol, both lowering your LDL level and increasing your HDL. These are the monounsaturated or polyunsaturated fats found in fish, nuts, and some vegetables. Olive oil and canola oil are examples of good fats.
   The bad fats are the saturated fats found primarily in red

meats and dairy products. Instead, think chicken, turkey, soy products, skim milk, and hard cheeses—rather than soft, high-fat varieties.

Trans fats are extremely bad fats, with a worse effect on your cholesterol and cardiovascular profile than any of the other kinds of fats. In the past, these lurked in the dark, unmentioned on food labels. Now, you can find them in nutrition labeling, as well as in ingredients lists as "partially hydrogenated" products. Fat that has been even partially hydrogenated is in fact totally bad. What the term means is that the fats are solid at room temperature—and what stays solid at room temperature is precisely what will clog your blood vessels at your body temperature. These fats are found mostly in such processed foods as desserts and snacks, and fast foods. One major indication of just how bad these fats are, is the FDA's Recommended Daily Allowance of trans fats in your diet: *zero*.

New, stricter requirements for food labels are prompting manufacturers to replace the trans fats in products with healthier alternatives. But remember that these processed or fried products probably still have the same number of calories as before, and are missing other healthy food components, so they should still rank as an occasional treat rather than part of your daily food pyramid. See chapter 8 on food for more details about fats.

2. **Again, try aerobic exercise.** This marvel of health improvement involves simply *moving your body* such that your heart rate is elevated, in whatever way you choose. Your lipids will be helped by this activity, while it also improves your insulin resistance, thus helping to lower your A1c, lower your blood pressure, and reduce your chance of heart disease. Resistance training, such as using bands or weights to tone your muscles, is also healthful when combined with aerobic exercise, but it is aerobic exercise that's king here (or queen, or just the jewel in the crown of exercise, if you will).

3. **Medications have become increasingly important in treating elevated lipid values as well.** The most important medications here are from a general family called **statins**, including lovastatins (Advicor, Mevacor, and Altocor), atorvastatins (Lipitor), and pravastatins (Pravachol and Pravigard). See chapter 11 for more details on these drugs.

   Advertised frequently on TV, statins really are very effective in reducing LDL, the most important lipid risk factor. Numerous clinical studies have actually shown that statins reduce both your chance of having a heart attack, and also from dying from a heart attack in case you do have one. In fact, these studies show that statins may have an additional cardiovascular health benefit separate from their effect on lowering LDL, helping to reduce inflammation of the lining of the arteries. Current studies are exploring this phenomenon more carefully.

4. **Reducing your A1c and carbohydrate intake can also be very useful for bringing down high triglycerides.**

If you are in debt, with LDL over 140, triglycerides over 400, and/or HDL less than 45

High LDL, and triglycerides in particular, put you at very high risk for heart disease. Here are the steps to take, starting with LDL, the most important risk factor of the three cholesterol values:

1. **If your LDL is greater than 140, your main approach will be the addition of a statin medication, or an increase in the dose of your present statin, or the addition of Zetia, a medication that can enhance the effect of the statins.** It is also crucial that you pay attention to the types of fat in your diet, altering your food choices if necessary to improve your LDL. Exercise will also aid in lowering your LDL but, at this level, the most important decreases will come from medication and dietary changes.

2. **If your triglycerides are greater than 400, you also have an elevated chance of developing pancreatitis, a painful and debilitating medical problem that can be difficult to treat.** Very high triglyceride levels may well be coupled with a high A1c value (the A1c does not have an impact on your LDL or HDL cholesterol, but it does have a big impact on your triglycerides). If your A1c is above 8.0, and particularly if it is over 9.0, then improvements in your glucose control will also result in improvements in your triglycerides. If you are eating high amounts of carbohydrate, reductions here can also reduce your triglycerides. In addition, reducing overall fat and eating better types of fat in your diet will also be very helpful.

   If your A1c is already in a reasonable range, and you're not overdoing carbohydrate intake, you will likely need medications to reduce your triglycerides. Some of the popular statins used to reduce LDL cholesterol can also decrease triglycerides, but you may need a *fibrate*, which works more specifically to reduce the triglycerides.

3. **The strategies to raise low HDL numbers (i.e., increase your "good" cholesterol) are going to sound familiar by now: aerobic exercise; attention to diet—especially adding soluble fiber in the form of oats, fruits, vegetables, and legumes; cutting trans fats; and stopping smoking.** (Soluble fiber is discussed in more detail in chapter 8). Studies show that it is also helpful to increase your intake of the "good" (monounsaturated, non-animal-derived) fats found in canola, avocado, or olive oil; nuts; and peanut butter. You might be surprised (even happy?) to hear that there is also good evidence that one or two drinks of alcohol per day (such as a glass of wine or beer) can significantly increase HDL levels—although the American Heart Association discourages doctors from advising patients to drink alcohol.

What Can You Do to Improve Your Microalbumin?

Lowering your microalbumin is almost always about lowering your blood pressure.

1. **Even if your blood pressure is on target, there are two classes of blood pressure medications that may help keep your kidneys safe and healthy: ACE inhibitors and ARBs, which have a directly protective effect on your kidneys, separate from their effect on lowering your blood pressure.** Both classes of drug work on the same kidney–blood-pressure pathway, but at different points, and taken together they have an *additive effect* (i.e., they are even more helpful together). A medication from one of these two classes is almost always the first choice in treating high blood pressure—thus lowering microalbumin—in patients with diabetes.

2. **Lower your blood pressure target. Even in the absence of diabetes, high blood pressure is one of the leading causes of kidney failure.** When diabetes is also present, you need to make sure that you are really hitting the target of below 130 systolic (upper number), and below 80 diastolic (lower number). In fact, if your microalbumin remains high after initial treatments, you should work to lower your systolic blood pressure to 125 or 120.

3. **Working to reduce your A1c, if it is high, will also help you achieve kidney health.**

If you are in debt, with microalbumin over 300

Microalbumin is a tricky test, so your first step here should be to repeat the test. If a second go confirms the high result, you should start directly on either an ACE inhibitor or ARB. If you are already taking one of these medications, you will need to increase the dose, and possibly add another medication. ACE inhibitors and ARBs work on the same general physiological pathway, but at different points, and clinical studies have shown that they are even more effective when taken together.

You should also move your systolic blood pressure target down to 125 or 120, depending on your present blood pressure and the degree of elevation of your microalbumin. You will need the advice of your doctor in both of these areas.

If your microalbumin remains high, consistently above 100, you should ask for a consultation with a nephrologist (a kidney specialist), to make sure that your treatment is optimized.

REAL PEOPLE:
RECOGNIZE YOUR TRUE HEALTH CHALLENGES

ELLIOTT, A SUCCESSFUL businessman in his mid-forties, was aware that his own diabetes care was lacking—especially in terms of diet—and wanted to do something about it. So he enrolled himself in a diabetes management seminar.

Naturally, part of this seminar was having participants tested for key health risk factors. Elliott's test results showed that everything was in pretty good range except his microalbumin, which was unacceptably high. The organizers discussed with him the meaning of microalbumin, and what he could do about it.

At the end of the four-day seminar, each participant was asked: "What's the one big thing you'll take away from this program in regard to your own health?" To which Elliott promptly replied, "I need to eat better."

The organizers were flabbergasted. Despite all the talk about test results and risk factors, Elliott was still fixated on the idea that he needed to revamp his diet. His high microalbumin result somehow didn't stick in his mind, although it posed a much more immediate health risk.

What Elliott really needed to take away from the seminar was a plan for addressing his microalbumin risk: first, to have the test repeated for accuracy; and then, if the results remained high, to see his doctor to determine if an additional ACE inhibitor medication could help.

Focus in on your true health risks, rather than on some general idea of healthier living not borne out by your test results.

What Can You Do to Improve Your Eye Health?

1. **Make sure you get an eye exam done regularly, preferably by an eye doctor who is especially familiar and practiced in the area of diabetic retinopathy.** Unfortunately, there's no easy way to assess your ophthalmologist's familiarity with diabetes. You can ask, and he or she may say something nondescript. You may need to be a bit pushy and insist that the doctor share information about his or her training and experience with diabetes-related eye disorders.

   In any case, the exam that this doctor conducts should include full dilation of your eyes. This is done by using drops that enlarge your pupils, making it easier for the ophthalmologist to see all parts of the retina in the back of your eyes. You should ask specifically if there are *any changes at all* in your eyes that may be related to your diabetes. Your doctor should also be able to supply you with a written report, so that you will be able to track your retina status over time. If you have any concerns about your eye exam, make an appointment with a retinal specialist; he or she should be able to supply you with the accurate information that you need. Specialized laser treatments to the retina are extremely successful (and painless) in stopping and sometimes reversing retinopathy.

   Patients who are screened appropriately are significantly less likely to develop eye disease in the course of their diabetes. As in most other areas, the sooner you start, the better your long-term outcome.

2. **You'll be happy to learn that improving your A1c can slow or reverse the progression of retinopathy and other eye problems.**

3. **Lowering your blood pressure, especially if it is elevated, can also be very helpful.**

If you are in debt, with proliferative retinopathy or macular edema

If eye problems have already developed, laser therapy is very effective, but you'll need to make careful choices. Unless you get your eye care at a health center that is known for specializing in diabetes, you should consider a second opinion, to help you make the best possible decision about the laser treatment you will likely need. As opposed to the other diabetes factors described here, you can't easily monitor your own eye status or determine the effectiveness of your treatment choices. For this reason, you want to be as confident as you can that your eye doctor is prescribing the optimal treatment.

Bringing down your blood pressure, if it is elevated, will also be extremely helpful here. If your A1c is high (over 9.0), you should specifically discuss your strategy for reducing it with your eye specialist as well as your regular doctor; in the case of advanced retinopathy, rapid changes in the A1c can sometimes lead to temporary worsening of the problem. But in the long run, reducing your A1c will have a strong positive impact on your eye health.

Overcoming Your Barriers

Now you know which steps you need to take to eliminate your health debts, and to start building up your health savings. Knowing where you stand is half the battle. Of course, actually implementing the necessary changes is the other half. In truth, we tend to discourage you from thinking about your diabetes as a battle, because that only makes you feel consistently at war with yourself—fighting off temptations left and right. Rather, we believe you can find a way to integrate your diabetes care into your life so that it doesn't cause constant anguish and you don't feel perpetually deprived.

Here are some approaches that may help:

Think of rewards, rather than punishment

People with diabetes often feel that things are being taken away from them. Try turning this around. Think about things you can do for your diabetes that also make you feel good, and be creative: find some ways to reward yourself for small accomplishments. For example, cutting out that second portion of potatoes at dinner and going for a walk every day can actually make you feel surprisingly good. Rather than flopping into bed with a full stomach, you feel lighter and more energetic in the mornings, and the regular walks will get you fresh air and keep you energized throughout the day.

Giving yourself little rewards when you reach incremental goals may also help motivate you. Some people pop a dollar bill in jar each time they go for a walk or a jog, for example. Use this booty to treat yourself to a massage or a pedicure or a new book or CD, whatever makes you happy. (Rewards shouldn't be edible.)

Remember how lucky you are: the diet and lifestyle changes you need to make for your diabetes can actually be pleasant and offer their own built-in rewards (unlike invasive treatments such as chemotherapy and dialysis). For example, it may be hard to get started with exercise, but once you do, you'll find that it reduces stress, boosts your mood, improves your body image, promotes a wonderful sense of well-being, and can even improve your sex life. Making the best of your diabetes care is all about your state of mind.

Doctors continuously note that the patients who do best with diabetes are the optimistic ones—not because they are by nature happy, but because optimism is really a problem-solving approach. When a bad thing happens to an optimistic person, that person feels empowered to do something about it. Pessimists, on the other hand, do not feel empowered, and compound the problem by telling themselves, "This will always happen to me." Instead, try telling yourself, "I did pretty good today."

Stop comparing yourself to others

Remember that people are at different stages in their diabetes care, so comparing yourself to others makes no sense. Think about the practical things you need to do to achieve your own goals. Are you on medications? Maybe you need more at this point. Or if your A1c is high, maybe you need to focus on overcoming your personal barriers to exercise, as discussed. Just because someone else seems fitter or on a better diet does not mean that you are failing. Conversely, just because someone else tried a particular medication and found it ineffective doesn't mean that it wouldn't work for you.

Your diabetes is unique, and your efforts to achieve good health are always worthwhile. Doing *something* is always better than doing nothing.

Create real strategies for your daily life

One of the most common barriers to good diabetes care seems to be the gap between the ideal advice patients get in the doctor's office, and what happens when they go out into the real world. We're all very busy and time seems to slip away as we chase after our own hectic schedules. Meanwhile, we often eat on the run, in places where the food choices are limited and far from the ideally healthful diet we'd like to follow. So it's important to strategize about overcoming obstacles in your daily routine:

What things usually get in the way of exercising, or eating better? And what can you do about them? What are some things you already spend time doing on a regular basis? Could you integrate some form of exercise into that activity, like taking a walk around the perimeter of the park while you wait for your child's soccer to practice to end? Or walking up the three flights of stairs to your office every morning instead of taking the elevator?

The goals you set should be behavioral: not a number, but rather something that you can actually do physically. For example, saying

"I'll lose ten pounds in the next three months" is not an achievable goal, because you cannot expressly control your weight. But you can control your eating. You can say, "I'm going to start adding more healthy vegetables to my dinner every night" or "I'll cut my down my junk food intake to a single portion of french fries per week. That'll be my weekend treat for eating healthfully all week."

Pace yourself and forgive mistakes

Overall, the two most important things you can do to make your diabetes care a natural part of your life—rather than some additional overwhelming burden—are pacing yourself and forgiving yourself.

Rather than beating yourself up about mistakes you've made, try to view your off-days and your off-target glucose results as information to help you decide what to do next. For example, if you ate three-quarters of a doughnut one day and your blood sugar shot up for the entire day, maybe next time you could eat just half the doughnut, and make sure you follow it up with a brisk walk.

In order to live at peace, you must accept that you cannot be the perfect patient all the time, because no one can spend every minute fussing about BG tests and never, ever eating off-limit foods. But you also cannot treat your diabetes like some crash diet: on again, off again, binging in between, and all the while torturing yourself with guilt. Guilt is really quite useless when it comes to diabetes. It shuts you down, stopping you from learning and from giving your best to take care of yourself every day.

So instead of trying to be perfect all the time, think about striving to do a pretty good job with your diabetes most of the time. This means doing the best that you can for your diabetes in every given situation, and also thoroughly forgiving yourself for slip-ups or bad days. What is key is letting the bad stuff go with enough finality that you feel ready to start over the very next day doing the best that you can, again. And so on. It means believing that your actions make a positive difference to your health, and not giving up.

How to Manage Your Health-Care Team: Take Control

ONE OF OUR main goals in writing this book is that, after reading it, you will no longer be entirely reliant on your doctor or educator. You yourself will know very well where you stand with your diabetes, and where you need to focus—which will make interaction with your health-care providers much more productive for both you and them.

You will know the results of your recent A1c test, your blood pressure, your triglycerides and cholesterol, your microalbumin sample, and your eye exam. You will also know whether you're able to balance your diabetes care reasonably well with the rest of your busy life—or if your present regimen is too overwhelming. You will know if diabetes is adversely affecting your personal life or your job, and will have learned ways to reduce those effects.

Of course, you will still need the help of medical professionals, because they have experience and expertise that is very useful for you. What we are saying is that by having a solid understanding of the present state of your diabetes, you will be ready to engage them at a new level—to help you troubleshoot problem areas, to obtain and maintain your goals, to answer all kinds of questions, and to inform you about new approaches, devices, or medications that may be helpful.

Getting the most out of your doctor appointments

Many people walk out of their doctor appointments feeling deflated, or sometimes even resentful. The best way to combat this frustration is to put yourself in control. Rather than passively waiting for the professionals to tell you what to do, you can walk in to the appointment prepared to ask for specific advice on areas that concern you.

The bulk of your diabetes care relies on you alone; only you can control it day-to-day. And your body will react differently to particular combinations of food, medications, and exercise than other people's do, so the traditional one-size-fits-all doctor's orders are not sufficient. It's up to you to act as team leader of your care team, guiding the members to provide the customized information and help that you need.

For example, let's say your A1c is above your goal, and you aren't sure what to do next. Maybe an increase in activity would be best, or maybe you could make further food changes; but these might be difficult with your current work schedule, or you may feel that you've already maxed out your efforts here, and just aren't getting results. So it might be that your diabetes itself is changing and you need a change in medication. Go into your appointment prepared to discuss your specific ideas—and pros and cons of approaches—with your doctor or diabetes educator.

Or perhaps your A1c is at your goal, but your blood pressure has consistently been in the 130s. Your care team, left to themselves, might simply be asking you the customary diabetes checkup questions about your BGs and losing weight. However, with your A1c at target, you know that the blood pressure is more of a risk factor for you, and you can direct the visit toward addressing this issue.

Think of your diabetes as a small business

To get you in the mindset of a take-charge approach, we recommend thinking of your diabetes as a small business, and your health-care team as your consultants. Again, the idea is to go into your appointments armed with information on where your "business" stands, and prepared with clear goals and/or questions they can advise you on. This way you won't end up just passively answering questions about how often you check your BG. Remember, these people work for you. Sometimes you might want an A1c test more often than every three months. If they push back on requests, it's your right as their client to insist, as well as to ask why they might be opposed to fulfilling your request at this time.

How to talk to your dietitian

What about a visit to a dietitian? These should be more helpful than they usually are. If you come in for the first time without
any specific questions or background information, you may get the
"daily special": you'll be informed of your ideal weight, handed a
calorie-restricted diet or a list of new, healthy foods to focus on, and
told how much to eat at each meal. Likely, none of these were reasons that you came to the appointment. Again, your goal should be
to utilize the dietitian as your consultant, so *you need to tell that
individual what it is you want to know*. Your purpose, especially for
an individual appointment, is not to hear a general lecture on diabetes and weight loss.

Your ultimate goal is to improve your long-term diabetes care and
overall health. So ask for information that will be truly useful in your
real-life, everyday routine. For most people, this means learning more
about the foods that they already eat regularly: What is the carbohydrate content of the ten or fifteen foods you eat most often?
What types of fat do they contain? You'll need to be aware of the
amounts you typically consume, and what foods you enjoy in situations where you can't read labels describing their components:
What's in pad thai, anyway? Carbs, fat, protein—how much? What's
the difference between Lemon Chicken and General Tso's Chicken?
What about burritos, and how can they vary? You get the idea.

By learning about foods you already eat, you'll be better able to
assess how your diet affects your A1c, lipids, and blood pressure.
You may find that you can make some positive changes simply by
eating *more* of some healthy foods you already like, while eating certain other foods less often.

If your LDL or HDL cholesterol are not at target, you'll want to
concentrate on the types of fat you're eating. Some fats can actually
help your cholesterol (although they still pack the same number of
calories), whereas some are especially harmful (think trans fats).

If your triglycerides are high (but your A1c is in a reasonable
range), you should also consider the amount of carbohydrates you're
eating. If you like to snack, and there are six different snacks you find

tasty, learn about them. Maybe three of these are a better fit with your diabetes than the others. Rather than adding completely new foods to your diet, it might be more practical to change the frequency or portion size of indulging in some foods that you already eat—in other words, keep eating what you like, but less of it.

This approach is especially useful in today's medical environment, when visits often seem rushed, and providers have a multitude of tasks to accomplish, many of them not directly related to your main concerns on that visit. If you wait until the end of the visit to bring up your specific concerns, you may run out of time. Instead, plan to ask your most pertinent questions as soon as you enter the room—maybe even before you sit down. By doing this, you will direct the discussion immediately toward your most useful path.

Make sure you see the results

We've hammered on the point that only by knowing the status of your own diabetes can you identify the areas where your doctor and health-care team can help you most. But once is not enough; *regular testing* is critical to your health, and to your motivation as well.

After the first round of tests, you may start out enthusiastic to make changes. But this can peter out fast. Without some kind of ongoing report card, you may begin to feel that your efforts are in vain. The idea is to keep updating copies of the chart in chapter 2. Place copies of your older and newer test results side by side, and compare the numbers. We encourage you to make copies of Your Diabetes Health Account, which also appears in the appendix of this book, that you can fill in, update, and keep handy for your own action plans and to bring along with you to appointments with your doctor or educators.

Just by focusing on an area for a few months, you will no doubt bring the test results closer to ideal range. You can see that you have made a difference. Hooray! It's good to know that your actions, not just your doctor's, are effective and make a big difference in your overall health.

Reward yourself in some positive way, and then set new goals for your next triumph. The ability to see the difference you have made is the key motivation for sticking to your new regimen. It's a rush, like working on your bank statement and discovering that there is much more money in the bank now than you had before.

If you do all this, there's no way for nasty complications to sneak up on you, because nothing ever happens suddenly with diabetes.

Crafting Your Plan

Now it's time to think about your own initial plan of action.

YOUR DIABETES CARE CYCLE

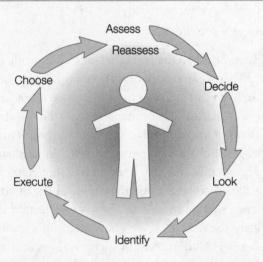

THINK OF TAKING care of your diabetes as a continuous cycle. You need to:

- **Assess your current results**
- **Decide what needs attention**
- **Look at your treatment choices (activity, food, medications)**

- Identify any stresses that are making your life more difficult
- Choose some appropriate actions
- Execute your actions, then
- Reassess your new results, and
- Cycle again through this circle of care

Remember also: There will be times when you are doing well, when your results are all in a safe range, and you won't need any immediate changes in your diabetes regime. But there will also be times when you feel like you're cycling uphill, and your diabetes care will require more intense effort. Push through these rough spots, and you will cycle back to another smooth stage.

Take a few moments now to do the following:

- Go back to chapter 2 to review your most urgent health debts. Even if you have several that need attention, it's wise not to tackle more than two at a time.
- Review the relevant sections in this chapter as a reminder of what you can do to improve on each area that needs work.
- Choose one or two strategies for each that you're willing to commit to. Think about some tactics for fitting these activities into your everyday life, so you can realistically stick with your plan.

For example, if you're committing to checking your glucose more often to help lower your A1c, maybe you can get a second meter to keep in your car or at your office, so you won't have to worry about forgetting it at home. Or if you're committing to taking your oral medications more religiously, you could buy a pill case that has slots for each day of the week, and keep it next to the kitchen sink, where you'll be sure to see it each morning.

YOUR ACTION PLAN

Improving Your A1c	Improving Your Blood Pressure	Improving Your Lipids	Improving your Microalbumin	Improving Your Eye Health
Choose Your Actions	**Choose Your Actions**	**Choose Your Actions**	**Choose Your Actions**	**Choose Your Actions**
• Exercise:	• Begin home monitoring:	• Eat fewer processed foods (reduce bad fats):	• Medication (ACE inhibitors and ARB's):	• Research eye doctors familiar with diabetes:
• Reduce carbohydrate intake:	• Medication(s):	• Eat more healthy fats:	• Control your blood pressure (lower your BP goal):	• Schedule annual eye exam:
• Reduce portion size:	• Exercise:	• Aerobic exercise:	• Other(s):	• Focus on improving A1c:
• Stress reduction tactics:	• Increase fruits and vegetables:	• Add or change medications		• Focus on reducing blood pressure:

Improving Your A1c	Improving Your Blood Pressure	Improving Your Lipids	Improving Your Microalbumin	Improving Your Eye Health
• Medication(s):	• Reduce salt intake:	• Other(s):	• Other(s):	• Other(s):
• Other(s):	• Other(s):			
Everyday tactics:	Everyday tactics:	Everyday tactics:	Everyday tactics:	Everyday tactics:
Notes:	Notes:	Notes:	Notes:	Notes:
Target date for next test:	Target date for next test:	Target date for next test:	Target date for next test:	Target date for next test:

4 Then What?
Setting the Tone for the Long Haul

What to Expect Over Time

ONE OF THE hallmarks of diabetes is its unpredictability. That is, whatever worked well for you last week or last month may not be doing the trick now. Sometimes you might go for a year or more on one regime, and suddenly start noticing that something's not right: you don't feel so well and your BG levels are less than desirable, confirmed by your A1c results. We must stress that this is not a sign of failure. In fact, it's perfectly normal that your diabetes will change over time. But as long as you know where you are, you can take action to get back on track immediately.

A good way to think about your day-to-day diabetes care is that it is like traveling. As you head down the road, you need to pay constant attention so you won't miss important turns or head the wrong direction.

Think of yourself armed with your glucose meter as a mountain climber with a compass. If you test your glucose and discover an off-target number, this is not a measure of your poor performance. Rather, the meter is a very useful tool to help guide you to where you need to go next. High or low numbers give you information on which way to turn. Over time, this might mean changing or adding medications, increasing your physical activity, altering your diet yet again, or addressing new stresses that have entered your life.

You can also think of the five key diabetes health tests introduced here as components of a GPS system (computerized navigation). Each component gives you information about where you need to take twists and turns for safe and successful driving. Without this information, you would certainly crash sooner or later.

Staying in the Driver's Seat

FOR THE MOMENT, hopefully you've addressed your most urgent health risks and turned these into health assets. Now, the important thing is not to fall asleep at the wheel. This is not a disease that can be handled on autopilot; you still have to keep a keen eye on the road ahead, because it will continue to change and bring on new challenges. This doesn't mean you need to maintain a state of crisis mode, just a state of clear awareness. By paying attention to your glucose level and the updated results of your five health tests, you will immediately notice if you begin to veer off target, and you'll know what to do in order to steer quickly back toward good health.

Returning to our banking analogy, you would do the same with your money in the bank, wouldn't you? Even if you'd paid off your immediate debts and got your finances in order, you wouldn't just forget about your savings and let them sit neglected for months or years. You know instinctively that you need to keep managing your money. You want your finances to stay healthy, with a goal of accumulating a nest egg of surplus money for later on when you need it most.

Whatever your metaphor, what this means in practical terms is that even if all five of your health factors are in the safe zone now, you need to continue having your tests done regularly. As a reminder:

- *every three months*—the A1c blood test
- *every six months at least*—blood pressure (have it checked

at every doctor's appointment if possible, especially if it's been a debt area)

- *annually*—microalbumin, lipids, and your eye exam (unless concerns call for more frequent checks)

Try to think about this as a simple matter of having a blood test four times a year, plus a urine and eye check once a year. That doesn't sound too bad, does it? The blood pressure is something you can have tested at every opportunity, even if you happen to be seeing your family doctor, gynecologist, dermatologist, or another physician for whatever reason; it takes just a moment to put the cuff on and take a reading. The imperative is that you record and understand your numbers, and stand ready to take action if you find that you're slipping into a "debt zone."

> REMEMBER, YOUR FIVE essential diabetes success factors are just like money in the bank. You wouldn't just let your life's savings sit neglected for long periods of time, would you?

Besides these essential tests, you will need to do *some* ongoing planning to keep up your diabetes health in your everyday life. For example, knowing that physical activity is an essential ingredient to long-term success, you'll want to have this in mind when you consider job changes, moving to a new town, or when planning a vacation. Are there places to walk? Will you be close to a gym? Will your new commute take up precious time that will make healthy eating and physical activity more difficult? Think about some options: could you walk around your office building on your lunch break, or pack healthy snacks in your car ahead of time, or arrange to go to a gym in the morning before work? These decisions are important for anyone concerned about his or her overall health and happiness.

When you have diabetes, those around you are also affected, which may not always be pleasant for them . . . and their concerns may come out in ways that are not helpful for you: *"Should you be eating that?" "You don't seem to be listening to me, maybe you should check your BG?"* Or perhaps people around you are making it harder for you to stick with the lifestyle changes you have made.

You need to find a way to blunt negative concerns and enlist people's assistance in a way that would be helpful to you. It's okay to be clear about questions you'd prefer they didn't ask. From your side, perhaps sharing some of your numbers would reassure them that you are on the right path. Perhaps they could also help support your lifestyle in little ways, like helping to keep the refrigerator stocked with diet drinks, not sabotaging your efforts by asking you to eat or "just taste" something you have declined, becoming your companion for daily walks, or helping the family find new, healthy snack foods to stock up on. Consider having them come with to your next health-care visit, to get a better understanding of diabetes treatment, and have their questions answered as well.

Remember that when your family and friends help you, they are helping themselves as well. If you feel better, they'll feel better. Plus, the activity and food choices important for diabetes are also very healthy choices for anyone, including people who do not have diabetes. If you have children, they share your genes, and consequently have a somewhat higher risk of future diabetes; studies show that regular physical activity and good food choices can decrease this risk by over 50 percent.

Of course, the thought of caring for your diabetes for the rest of your life can seem daunting. But thinking about it this way may help remove some of the dread: it's just another practical area—like your financial security—that you want to manage as well as you possibly can to ensure a brighter future.

REAL PEOPLE:
DO WHAT YOU CAN

FREDERICK, A MIDDLE-AGED man with type 2 diabetes, came into the clinic utterly frustrated: His A1c was too high, and he was struggling terribly in trying following the recommended diet. Even the changes he did manage to make didn't seem to lower his glucose levels one bit. What could he do?

As it turned out, Frederick was a chef in an upscale New York restaurant, where he was surrounded by rich foods he was expected to prepare and taste day in and day out. No wonder the bland diet he'd been given didn't work for him.

The team at the diabetes clinic had a frank discussion with Frederick about what was realistic, given his life. What *else* was he willing to do in order to put some more savings in his diabetes health account, other than struggling to stick to his diet?

It turned out that he was amenable to starting an exercise regimen, and the team also added an oral medication to help further reduce his glucose levels. Shortly after making these changes, Frederick's A1c came down to a healthy level and has stayed there ever since.

Frederick was simply delighted to learn that there were other paths to reaching his health goal. Initially, he was so discouraged about his food issues and test results that he felt like giving up. But he learned that he could choose actions that actually fit his daily lifestyle. This more realistic strategy had a huge motivational benefit, too, because it's always easier to make small adjustments to your health regime once your numbers are already in range and you're feeling encouraged and empowered.

Taking on unrealistic goals that make you feel like you're constantly failing is totally unproductive.
Choose actions that you can make and stick with.

Overcoming Frustration:
Bumps in the Road

WITHOUT A DOUBT, diabetes can be terribly frustrating at times. It's fine to acknowledge your exasperation periodically, as long as you don't make your diabetes synonymous with frustration. Think of your bad days as bumps in the road. Of course, you'll hit a bad patch now and then, but this doesn't mean you're a bad driver, and with a little concentrated steering, you'll be back on smooth road again very soon.

People often refer to experience with a disease as a battle, such as "her battle with cancer," "his battle with leukemia," and so on. We think this reference is wholly inappropriate for diabetes—one of the few chronic diseases with which patients have the power to both feel physically well day to day, and to live a long and healthy life.

It is not at all helpful to think of diabetes as a war you have to win, because you yourself become the enemy. The battle turns into your "good" and well-behaved self versus your "evil" natural temptation to slack off or eat forbidden foods. This approach of being constantly at war with yourself will make you feel miserable and hopeless. What you must do, on the other hand, is accept that your diabetes is a lifelong condition that, if well controlled, can run parallel with the rest of your lifestyle. To keep it parallel and avoid a collision course (the battle scenario) requires you to be diligent about certain actions: taking medicine, eating healthfully and in moderation, and exercising. You can find a way to accomplish these things without hating yourself each time you let yourself down.

If you love greasy fast food, for example, maybe you can allow yourself one item per week. Perhaps you splurge every Sunday and eat a bag of french fries or onion rings. As long as you're eating healthfully the rest of the week, this shouldn't be a major problem, and it could be beneficial if it helps you feel less deprived most of the time. Rather than suffering from unfulfilled cravings every day, you can look forward to your weekly treat.

FRUSTRATION SAPS YOUR positive energy, making you less able to care for yourself. If you think of your diabetes as a battle, you'll always be stuck in a miserable war. Make peace with your diabetes, and you'll be at peace with yourself.

Finding Your Own Motivation

THINK ABOUT WHAT matters in your life. Are you on the path to a high-level career? Working to generate energy for your children or grandchildren? Hoping to enhance your relationship with your partner or spouse? Whatever it is, it's not going to happen unless you make taking care of your diabetes about *you*. You have to be making healthful food and exercise choices and taking your medications not because your doctor said so, or even because your family's pestering you, but because *you care about your own health and believe that your actions matter*. Wise diabetes experts say: "Do it for yourself first, and then enjoy the benefits for all."

Also take note that pleasure in succeeding is essential to your continued success. But your expectations have to be realistic. You can find pleasure in gradual change, such as a small improvement in your A1c, or being able to exercise a few minutes more today than you could do last week, or the week before. It's also helpful to think in terms of goals and rewards. Again, you'll want to keep it humble. A goal might be to jog past the first park bench to the second one tomorrow. A way to reward yourself for a job well done might be getting a massage or a pedicure, or buying a new book or CD. You might try sticking a dollar in a jar each time you exercise. Once you've gathered $25 or more, you have a little extra cash to treat yourself to something nice. (Remember: rewards shouldn't be edible.)

If you've tried changes in one area that don't seem to yield results, maybe it's time to move on. Try tackling another area of your lifestyle that may be easier for you to change. Again, your body does change over time, so it's not unusual to find that what worked last year is no longer working this year. If you accept that success with diabetes is an ongoing process, you'll be less frustrated at having to "start over" now and then.

Outliving Diabetes with Happiness and Success

HERE ARE A FEW enduring truths to keep in mind when it comes to pursuing a long and enjoyable life with diabetes:

- It's true that diabetes never goes away, and the underlying disease process continues over time. This doesn't mean that you are going to suffer complications, but rather that you may need to change your approach in response as time goes on.
- You'll need to monitor your five health factors regularly, *and* follow your BG levels regularly.
- It's essential for you to make regular physical activity a major priority.
- You should become an expert on the foods you like— what is the carbohydrate, fat, fiber, and calorie content of your most commonly eaten foods? What do they do to your BG? Trial-and-error can teach you a lot about which foods you might need to limit or counteract with a brisk walk after eating.

The happy ending is knowing that if you do all this, there's no way for nasty complications to sneak up on you, because nothing ever happens suddenly with diabetes. Complications are the outcome of long years of poor health management, which this book teaches you to avoid. By now you should know that you can *outlive* your diabetes happily and successfully.

5

Test Details:
All You Want to Know and More

NOW YOU KNOW your five key tests and why they're so important to your health. But if our brief introduction didn't tell you all you want to know about these life-sustaining examinations, then read this chapter to be more precisely informed.

A1c: Best Measure of Your Glucose Control

BY NOW YOU should know that the A1c is the single most important test reflecting your BG control, offering an average of BG values over the last several months. All of the clinical and basic research studies point to this test as the major indicator of future risk for diabetes-related complications. Despite its primary importance, fewer than 10 percent of patients with diabetes are aware of their last A1c result.

A1c is a short name for "glycosylated hemoglobin A1c." *Glycosylation* describes a process in which glucose molecules stick to proteins after being exposed to them over a period of time. *Hemoglobin* is a large molecule that is present in your red blood cells. Its major purpose is to pick up oxygen in your lungs and carry the oxygen to your body's cells. Over time, glucose molecules in your blood will stick, or become irreversibly attached, to the hemoglobin molecule, as they do to many proteins. The more glucose present in your blood, the more it becomes attached to your hemoglobin molecules. Measuring the amount of glycosylation of hemoglobin, rather than the glycosylation of other proteins, is useful in diabetes for two reasons:

1. **The hemoglobin protein is easily accessible for testing, simply by drawing blood.** Measuring glycosylation of other proteins such as those in your liver or the cells of your blood vessels might be useful and interesting for study, but also quite difficult and painful.

2. **The life of your red blood cells is fairly short.** Your red blood cells undergo a lot of wear and tear and survive, on average, for about 100 to 120 days, after which they are broken down and replaced. If your red blood cells never broke down, measuring the glycosylated hemoglobin would reflect your average BGs for your lifetime. Because of their constant breakdown and replacement, however, they reflect your average BGs over the last three to four months. This is a very practical timeframe in which to get an accurate assessment of your average BGs, similar to a quarterly report.

How the measurements are done

Historically, the A1c test was very confusing because different laboratories had different ways of going about measuring glycosylated hemoglobin—examining different subtypes of the hemoglobin using different laboratory techniques. So results not only differed, but were next to impossible to compare.

Fortunately, the American Association of Clinical Chemistry (AACC) established a subcommittee in 1993 to standardize A1c tests. A standard protocol was completed in 1996, and the National Glycohemoglobin Standardization Program (NGSP) was established to implement the new standard. It is now easier to understand your result, and to compare it to your previous result, regardless of which laboratory you use. The gold standard of measurement, used in all clinical trials involving A1c measures to date, here and around the world, is called high performance liquid chromotography (HPLC).

Since many local laboratories do not actually use HPLC, even now, the NGSP officially certifies different measurement techniques as reproducible, and traceable to the HPLC A1c standard. Thus laboratories using different approaches can report their results, corrected to the same standard, so that you can compare your results from different labs. One way to check on this is to look at the normal range for the lab reporting your result. It should be close to 4.0 to 6.0, which is the ideal range for people without diabetes.

Testing types and frequency

The A1c test is a blood analysis. If you are unsure about an A1c test that you have had at a new lab, you can always request that the sample be measured using the true HPLC technique. Even if not available in the local lab, they will be able to send it to a centralized lab where this method is available.

Usually this test is conducted in a lab setting, but a few companies have come out with A1c home testing kits in the last few years. These are mail-in laboratory tests, allowing you to draw your own blood using your lancing device at home, and then mail in the test card for results. This way, you get medical lab accuracy from the privacy of your own home. You can purchase these kits over the counter or directly from the manufacturers, including Diabetes Technologies Inc. (www.diabetestechnologies.com), BioSafe Laboratories (www.ebiosafe.com), and Flexsite Diagnostics, Inc. (www.flexsite.com). Multiple test cards retail for around $25.

Wherever and however it is performed, this test reflects your average BGs over the last three to four months. So you should have your A1c checked at least every three months. Even if your BGs seem steady and you are following a successful regimen, the only way to really know where you stand over time is to know your A1c result.

Although the A1c looks backward over a period of months, half of the impact upon it comes from the last month. This means that sometimes it is useful to have your A1c tested more often. If you have started a new exercise program, made some significant changes in your food choices, or changed your medication, you can recheck your A1c in as early as one month's time to make sure that you are moving in the right direction.

Blood Pressure: Hypertension Detector

HIGH BLOOD PRESSURE is sometimes called *hypertension*. This term can be misleading, since high blood pressure is not a direct measure of being tense or having a high degree of tension in your life. Although stressful situations may sometimes (but not always) elevate your blood pressure, feeling calm and healthy is no guarantee that you do not have high blood pressure. Although some people believe they can detect when their blood pressure is high based on the way they feel, this is rarely the case. Your blood pressure needs to be extremely high, usually higher than 200/100, before you can feel symptoms.

FEELING GOOD ≠ GUARANTEED GOOD HEALTH

THE DISPARITY BETWEEN how you feel and your test results holds true for all the tests discussed in this book.

You might feel great, even when your A1c, blood pressure, lipids, microalbumin, or retinal condition are way out of your target range.

Conversely, you may feel tired, depressed, have pain or other discomforts, even while all these tests are in a good range.

The only way to really know where you stand—with regard to your risk of future diabetes-related complications—is to be tested regularly, and take the time to review and compare the results.

That being said, blood pressure does vary throughout the day, often going up with exertion and stress. Some people do experience higher blood pressures at their health-care provider's office than they do at other times. This increase, called "white coat hypertension," is not totally benign, however. Research studies have shown that people experiencing this type of doctor-associated hypertension also have an increased risk of heart attacks and strokes. This makes sense, as being stressed out over a doctor's appointment is an indicator of how your body reacts to other, frequent stresses: most of us regularly experience situations at least as stressful as visiting our doctor many times throughout a typical day, perhaps without being as overtly conscious of that tension.

Testing types and frequency

You should have your blood pressure checked whenever you visit a clinic or health-care facility. If it is above target, no need to panic. Have it checked again within the next two months to confirm. If you are taking blood pressure medication or if your blood pressure is just barely at or under your target, it may be helpful to do home blood pressure monitoring using a portable home monitoring device as well, checking once or twice a week. Your blood pressure should be the same in both arms, so use whichever is most convenient (unless you have had lymph gland removal in one arm, as a result of such procedures as a mastectomy, in which case you should use the other arm exclusively). Write down the results in the same log book that you use to record your BG results.

Note, however, that many home devices are not accurate, particularly the ones that attach to your wrist or finger. Unfortunately, many of the machines placed for public use in pharmacies and retail stores are also inaccurate. Ask your health-care provider for a recommendation of a reliable home blood pressure monitor, and take it with you to several health-care provider visits, so that you can compare your results to those in the medical office. Some gyms will also have onstaff exercise physiologists who have the right training and equipment to provide you with accurate results.

If you measure your blood pressure after sitting quietly for ten minutes, the result should almost always meet the target of less than 130/80. If you are checking your blood pressure at home, a good time to conduct the test is in the morning after you've been awake for a short while. In rare cases where your blood pressure results are highly variable, you may need to wear a 24-hour blood pressure monitor to get an accurate reading. Usually, however, this is not necessary.

Don't forget to write the numbers down so that you can review them yourself later, and discuss them with your doctor. Basing a decision on eight or more numbers, spread throughout a month, will be much more useful than making therapy changes based on just two results obtained in the doctor's office one month apart.

Lipids: Cholesterol Barometer

THIRTY YEARS AGO, most of us never hear of cholesterol. But this has become a household word for Americans middle-aged and beyond. Clinical studies in the 1970s linked high total cholesterol to heart disease, but it would be years before the hypothesis was confirmed that lowering cholesterol, by whatever means, also lowers your chance of heart disease and stroke. It took many more years and many clinical studies to begin to tease out the different components of the total cholesterol measurement.

Nowadays, three different lipid components are routinely measured; LDL cholesterol, HDL cholesterol, and triglycerides. Since the LDL cholesterol is the most difficult to measure, most lab tests take direct measures of your total cholesterol, HDL cholesterol, and triglycerides. The LDL value is then calculated by using the following formula:

LDL = total cholesterol − HDL cholesterol − triglycerides/5

This calculated LDL is often reported as LDL(c), and is fairly accurate as long as the triglyceride result is below 400.

Although the total cholesterol is sometimes mentioned as a risk factor, it is no longer considered useful, given the easy availability of the more specific and more informative LDL, HDL, and triglyceride tests. For example, a total cholesterol of 173 could be just as easily associated with very healthy cholesterol results (LDL 80, HDL 65, triglycerides 140) as with very unhealthy results (LDL 140, HDL 25, triglycerides 40). Therefore a total-cholesterol measurement doesn't tell you much about your health.

As mentioned in chapter 2, LDL and HDL cholesterols are not affected by meals, but your triglyceride level does rise directly after you've eaten. Nevertheless, it is not usually necessary to have your tests conducted when you're fasting, unless you've had an elevated triglyceride result and are concerned.

Testing types and frequency

There are no accurate home monitors for cholesterol available at this time, but there are some products in the pipeline. Meanwhile, you will need to obtain a lab order from your health-care provider and visit the medical lab to have your blood drawn. If you have started on a new regimen to control your abnormal lipid values, such as food changes, increased activity, or a medication change, you should be able to see the results within six weeks. If your lipid results are meeting your target, testing once a year is reasonable. Exceptionally good lipid results need be repeated only every two years, unless there is a change in lifestyle or medication. Of course, if your lipid values are this good, you may want to hear the good news more than once every two years.

Microalbumin: Early Detector of Kidney Disease

CLINICAL STUDIES REPEATEDLY show that this is the test least often done in patients with diabetes, which is a shame, because it's such a powerful tool. In the past, the early stages of kidney failure were not detectable in patients with diabetes. The best tests available were either measuring creatinine in the blood, or a crude measure of the total protein content in the urine. Changes in these test results only show up relatively late in the process of kidney disease, therefore by the time damage was identified, end-stage kidney failure would usually occur within the next ten years. At that late stage, patients were usually unable to prevent the eventual loss of kidney function.

In the 1970s, researchers began to develop methods to measure much smaller amounts of protein in the urine, in particular albumin, the most common protein in the blood. Eventually, they were even able to detect very small amounts—micrograms even—of this protein in the urine. This ability gave the test the name *microalbumin*. In contrast, the old urine protein test was only able to detect protein amounts in the high milligram and gram level. You can appreciate the enormous increase in sensitivity of the microalbumin test by considering the fact that there are a thousand micrograms in a milligram, and a thousand milligrams in a gram.

How the measurements are done

Testing for various substances in the urine is actually pretty tricky. It is always complicated by the variable volume and concentration of the urine supplied. Although in general, urine secretion of albumin is fairly constant, the amount of microalbumin in a single urine specimen is quite variable. If only a short amount of time has passed since the bladder was last emptied, then there will only be a small amount of microalbumin present. This variability can be corrected by dividing by the volume of urine, to provide the *concentration* of microalbumin. This allows samples from small volumes of urine to be compared to samples from larger volumes of urine. But this still doesn't account for the fact that urine is more concentrated during some time periods than others, depending on how much fluid the patient has drunk.

For these reasons, many urine collections for medical purposes use the total urine collected during a 24-hour period. While more exact, this method is much more cumbersome for patients. Of course you can try to schedule your "collection" for a weekend, but sometimes you still might end up carrying around a urine collection container all day, in your car or in your office refrigerator. You can imagine the potential for mishaps.

Fortunately, an elegant solution has been found for this problem. Your body, unbeknownst to you, secretes a protein called creatinine, at a very constant rate. By measuring the creatinine level along with the albumin level in a single urine sample, the lab is able to accurately determine the excretion level of albumin. This test is aptly called the microalbumin/creatinine ratio. This ratio gives results that are just as accurate as the burdensome 24-hour collections. Some labs routinely measure and/or report only the microalbumin results, however, and not the microalbumin/creatinine ratio. Whenever your results are a little high, you should ask for the more sensitive and more specific ratio test.

Testing types and frequency

As discussed above, you should ask to have this test conducted on a single urine sample, correcting for creatinine, the so-called urine microalbumin/creatinine ratio. If your results have been in the normal range (usually less than 30), then once a year is fine for frequency of testing.

If you have had a high result, hopefully you are taking steps to improve it: taking an ACE inhibitor, an ARB, controlling your blood pressure, and/or improving your A1c. In this case, you will want to monitor the microalbumin/creatinine ratio more often to determine the success of your treatments, and in order to decide whether you need to add something new to your current approach.

Eye Exam: Test for Healthy Retinas

THE EYE EXAM is the most difficult test for you to judge, since your ophthalmologist does not usually give you a precise grading of your eye status. Usually, you'll hear that your eyes are either "okay" or that you need to have treatment such as laser therapy. This can be a bit disconcerting, so don't hesitate to ask your doctor for a more detailed explanation.

Eye exams are usually performed by either optometrists or ophthalmologists, but you want to insist on the latter. Optometrists are certified after attending four years of optometry school following college. They deal primarily with routine exams and fitting corrective lenses. Ophthalmologists are the medical doctors who have received three or more years of specialty training following their four years of medical school. They perform eye surgery (cataract removals being the most common), and also use lasers to treat problems in the retina (the area in the back of your eye where light is detected). These are the folks best qualified to conduct a diabetes-related eye exam.

The most worrisome diabetes-related eye changes, retinopathy and macular edema, both occur in the retina, and are related to the duration and success of your diabetes control. Note that neither will cause visual changes until they are very advanced. This is why regular eye exams are so important. You probably won't notice anything until it's too late. Only a trained ophthalmologist providing a proper eye screening can detect damage early on. If you are screened regularly, chances are that any new changes in your vision won't be results of retinopathy or macular edema, but rather short-term swings in your glucose levels or age-related changes.

Testing types and frequency

If your eyes show no changes or minimal changes, then a dilated-eye exam once a year is sufficient. However, if your eyes show more advanced changes in your retina, your ophthalmologist will ask you to return much sooner, so that any required treatments can be started directly. This usually means laser treatment, targeting the areas of change in your retina. Luckily, laser surgery is extremely effective in treating diabetic retinopathy.

Your yearly eye exam will be able to detect other eye concerns also, including non-diabetes-related changes (e.g., macular degeneration), some changes which are slightly more common in diabetes (cataracts), and some changes whose relation to diabetes is unclear (glaucoma).

Along with the other four tests, you'll want a written record of your results. This is much less common, but your eye doctor is required to provide a report upon your request. This way you will have a better idea of your results, be able to note changes over time, and also be able to supply the results to your other health-care providers, rather than relying on the medical offices to communicate with each other. (Informal surveys reveal that when patients request results to be sent from one medical office to another, the likelihood of success is less than 50 percent.)

Meticulous Clinical Studies Support the Magic Five

WHILE WE'RE IN the midst of explaining the medical details, this is a good opportunity to point out that we're not making this stuff up. Over the last fifteen years, multiple, large, prospective, randomized, controlled, blinded clinical studies have explored the impact of these five tests and future diabetes-related complications. Because these clinical trials have been so important, you might be interested in taking a brief look at what all the terms mean, because this helps to explain their importance. In essence, these are all provisions to ensure that the study results are unbiased and fully credible.

Prospective means that the studies were planned before the occurrence of the events that they measured, compared to *retrospective* studies, which are conducted to look backward and explore events that have already occurred.

Controlled means that there is second group of subjects, similar to those who were treated, but who didn't receive the primary treatment. You need them so you can compare the results of the two groups to better understand what the effects of the treatment were. For instance, if you followed a group of people treated with a pink pill for ten years, you might find that they gained an average of ten pounds. Is this weight gain a direct effect of the pink pill? If you also followed a *control group*, that didn't receive the pink pill, you might find that their average weight gain was twenty pounds. Now, your conclusion might be very different; it seems that the pink pill might help people keep their weight down. Of course, for the control comparison to be most useful, the groups must be comparable in all risk factors that are important to the topic being studied. For example, here you would want to know that the same number of people in each group live next to a doughnut shop, or that equal numbers were active members of fitness centers.

Randomizing study groups means that a computer program randomly assigns individuals to either the treatment group, or the control group. This compensates for any unknown risk factors that you might not have recognized. Perhaps people with blue eyes are more likely to gain weight than are people with brown eyes, and since you are attracted to people with blue eyes, you might unknowingly assign more of them to the study group than the control group. Randomizing eliminates this possibility.

Blinding (or sometimes called *masking*) adds another layer of protection from biased results. The idea is that research subjects do not actually know if they are receiving the treatment, or if they are part of the control group. In our example above, the control group also takes a pink-colored pill, but one that is a placebo, i.e., contains no active ingredient. In what is called a *double-blind* study, even the researchers don't know who's receiving the real treatment, until the end of the trial, when the "code" is broken, and the data is analyzed.

Because it is difficult to perform a large-scale, long-duration, prospective, randomized, controlled, double-blinded clinical trial, lots of research uses less rigorous approaches. This is one of the reasons why news reports of research seem confusing and contradictory; does coffee hurt your health or help it? And what about alcohol? Many studies suggest that moderate alcohol consumption may decrease heart problems. But no one really knows, and it is unlikely that we will soon be able to identify large numbers of people in their forties or fifties who don't drink, and then randomly assign some to moderate alcohol consumption for the next five to ten years, and others to total abstinence. Blinding the study would be even more difficult: how could some people drink alcohol without knowing it? You get the idea; some questions are difficult to answer with certainty through clinical studies.

But regarding the impact of A1c, blood pressure, lipids, microalbumin, and eye exams, the answers are much more clear. There *have* been large-scale, long-duration, prospective, randomized, controlled double-blinded (with some exceptions where blinding was difficult) trials that confirmed the powerful effects of controlling these factors. Moreover, there weren't just one or two or even three studies in each area, but multiple studies, all supporting the same conclusions.

The conclusions are: keeping these five key factors in a safe range will ensure that you have reduced or even eliminated your chance of diabetes-related future health complications.

TWO LANDMARK STUDIES
THAT CHANGED THE DIABETES WORLD

- **THE DIABETES CONTROL AND COMPLICATIONS TRIAL (DCCT)**—the world's first large-scale, comprehensive diabetes study. From 1983 to 1993, the National Institute of Diabetes and Digestive and Kidney Diseases (NIDDK) tracked 1,441 volunteers with *type 1 diabetes* across twenty-nine medical centers in the United States and Canada. Volunteers had diabetes for at least one year but no longer than fifteen years. They also were required to have no, or only early signs of, diabetic eye disease.

  This study provided the first-ever concrete evidence that keeping blood glucose levels as close to normal as possible slows the onset and progression of eye, kidney, and nerve diseases caused by diabetes. It actually demonstrated that any sustained lowering of blood glucose helps, even if the person had a history of poor glucose control.

- **THE UNITED KINGDOM PROSPECTIVE DIABETES STUDY (UKPDS)**—in the largest clinical research study of diabetes ever conducted, the Diabetes Research Laboratories at Oxford followed over 5,000 patients with *type 2 diabetes* in twenty-three clinical centers based in England, Northern Ireland and Scotland for twenty years. Results were reported in 1998.

  This study provided the first conclusive evidence that the life-threatening complications of type 2 diabetes—diabetic eye disease, kidney damage, heart attacks, and strokes—can be significantly reduced via tight control of blood glucose and blood pressure.

These two studies form the springboard for today's more intense—and infinitely more successful—diabetes therapy.

6

Glucose Monitoring

Why You Need to Do It

WHY IS IT so important to check your BG? We've heard many people say, "My BG levels are high all the time. I already know that!"

That may be true for the time being, but your BG does fluctuate—even throughout the day—and there are at least a half-dozen good reasons for you to monitor it closely.

We've just finished explaining in great detail the five tests that tell you where you stand with your diabetes and your personal risk of developing future problems. The A1c test is the one that best reflects your BG levels by providing a three-month average. While the A1c and your daily BG measurements are obviously related, you need to view them as distinct entities, with the understanding that they provide you with very different types of information.

Information You Can Act On

REMEMBER WE SAID that if the question is "What effect are my BG levels having on my chance of future complications?" the answer is

"What is my A1c?" But if your A1c turns out to be above your target, this test doesn't provide a clue as to what you can do about it. A high A1c result only tells you that you need to change *something*.

On the other hand, it is your individual daily glucose results that can suggest specific actions or strategies. For example, you might notice that you tend to get very high readings after breakfast, whereas your late afternoon levels are not nearly as high. This would give you a tip to consider changing your breakfast menu and/or to schedule your exercise midday in order to bring your glucose levels down. Addressing these problem areas will of course improve your control over time and bring down your A1c result by your next test.

Also, since the A1c test is done intermittently, only every three months or so, checking your own BG regularly gives you a different sort of information, tied much more closely to your daily and weekly routine. This information falls into four different categories, each of which is very useful. Your BG readings can:

1. Provide short-term information about your BG control, and whether it has changed.
2. Show you the effects of your exercise.
3. Demonstrate the effects of specific foods and meals.
4. Tell you whether your BG is too low.

In addition, for patients who take insulin, you may need the BG readings to make daily adjustments in your insulin dose.

Perhaps the most important reason to check your BG is that checking it regularly can tell you if you are hitting your general BG targets, and obtain *early warning* about changes in your overall BG control.

What Should Your Targets Be?

You may not be exactly clear on where your BG numbers should be. The traditional targets are less than 130 before meals, and less

than 180 after meals. We believe that these ideal numbers are mis-
named "targets"; they are better viewed as "normal" readings that
people without diabetes experience almost all the time, and not
necessarily as useful targets for people with diabetes.

Setting targets that you know you will miss repeatedly is not very
helpful, especially when these targets are not directly linked to
reducing future risk. (These targets can certainly be useful in
increasing someone's diabetes stress, however, as in having your
partner remark, "What?! Why are you so high before lunch??")

This brings us to another fundamental (and somewhat quirky)
difference between your A1c and your daily glucose targets: many
patients with diabetes can meet their A1c target, while missing
these before- and after-meal targets frequently. What does this
mean? Remember that the A1c in an *average* number, in other
words a point that reflects the "middle" of all your glucose values
in the past three months. So you could have a perfect A1c result
of 6.5 that might actually reflect the midpoint between several
weeks of severe highs and lows (below 70). Not good.

If, however, your A1c met your target, and you *did not* have frequent low BG values, then all of your levels during the previous
three months were okay. They were okay even if they occasionally
fell out of the target ranges mentioned above, and okay even if you
sometimes had numbers over 200 that frustrated you. This is an
important point. You do need the information that daily glucose
monitoring provides, but you cannot and need not beat yourself up
over occasional "bad" numbers. There will always be fluctuations,
which is why the A1c is the perfect complement to daily testing.
Read on for the explanation.

Cut Daily Monitoring Stress with Your A1c

DIABETES COMES WITH enough of a regular hassle: sticking your
fingers to check your BG, thinking about what you eat, trying to
exercise regularly, worrying about the future. You don't want to add

needless frustrations. So stop stressing over every imperfect number you see on your glucose meter. If your A1c is on target, you have met your goal of bringing your BG levels into a safe range, therefore successfully decreasing your chances of glucose-related complications in the future. You were successful even if some of your daily readings were higher than the traditional targets, or higher than you liked.

Obviously your A1c and your daily BG results are linked, because the A1c provides an integrated value over the last several months. But the average of the BG values you've taken with your meter will not correlate perfectly with your A1c. This is mostly due to the fact that you are only checking several times a day, rather than hundreds, and that the times you check are not random, but rather the times most useful for your specific diabetes treatment regimen. You may tend to check regularly after eating, for example, when your glucose will inevitably be high. This is fine.

The point to remember is that individual BG numbers are not associated with complications, and hitting or missing these daily targets does not foretell your future. All of the existing clinical research tells us that your A1c is the vital indicator of your future health.

> **YOUR BG READINGS** do not serve the same purpose as your A1c. Your daily readings help you make daily choices. Your A1c tells you how you are doing overall.

All Glucose Readings Are Good

THIS BRINGS UP another important point, which is that *every BG check you do is good*—good in the sense that if you hadn't checked, you wouldn't have that information. Let's say for example you have a BG of 240 at bedtime; not a bad number, just a number. In fact, an interesting number. If you hadn't checked, you wouldn't know that you were high at bedtime. What does this tell you? Well, perhaps you rarely check at bedtime. Now you know that this may be a noteworthy time for you. If your A1c has been above your goal, perhaps it is because your late evening numbers are high. You might want to think about what you're doing in the evenings that may be causing that rise, such as regularly eating too many high-carb choices as part of your dinner.

Or, let's say you have that same 240 at bedtime, and you do know that this is higher than your usual bedtime numbers. Now you can think briefly about whether your supper meal and evening activities were different than usual. Did you eat different foods? Or sit very still while watching TV instead of straightening up the garage while listening to the Red Sox on the radio? Or did you grab some extra snacks tonight? If you can't identify any reasons for the higher value, let it go. Patterns of BG changes generally make sense, but single results often don't. What is important is that an occasional high BG incident causes no immediate damage to your body, even if it remains elevated for a while. Diabetes-related complications are never brought on by just one value, but rather over lengthy periods of time, which is reflected by an increased A1c (and high A1c values over years).

"GLUCOSE CHECKING" VERSUS "TESTING"

NOTE THAT YOU want to "check" your BG and not "test" it. If you are reading this book, it's very likely that you are the type of person who will want to "pass" every diabetes-related test you take.

Remember that your daily BG values aren't a test that you're going to pass or fail. Rather, they are information that helps you to improve your long-term control, which is measured with the A1c. If there were a test at which you want to excel, it would be the A1c, along with the other four assessments we've introduced in this book.

Get Practical Help with Lows, Food, and Exercise

IT MIGHT BE inconvenient, but it's also very practical to check your BG regularly, as it can give you early warnings about changes in your overall glucose control. If your glucose values are usually in the 140 to 180 range, but you began to see more numbers over 200, this will alert you that it's time to reassess your present regimen. This could mean that your diabetes itself is changing and that you may need a change in medication. The higher numbers could also reflect a change from your usual lifestyle choices, either in food or activity. Or perhaps you are not taking your medication as regularly as before.

Most current meters have the ability to store hundreds of glucose values, and show a running two-week average of your BG numbers. If you usually check your glucose at about the same times each day, changes in this fourteen-day average can remind you to look at your diabetes regimen a little more carefully. If this average remains high, you should request an A1c test for a more exact look at whether there has been a significant change.

Newer meters also display the time and date, enabling you to write your glucose results down in a diabetes log to look for patterns. Your doctor or diabetes educator may ask you to do this for certain periods in order to observe your routine. Obviously, relying on the meter only works when you have remembered to correctly enter the date and time. Check your meter manual or the company Web site for instructions on how to do this. You can also look up how to set alarms on your meter to remind you to check your glucose at certain intervals if you wish.

YOUR METER'S MEMORY
OFFERS A "PROGRESS REPORT"

MOST GLUCOSE METERS allow you to easily check your average BG for the last seven, fourteen, and sometimes even thirty days. This offers a great "progress check" if you've started a new exercise program, or your partner has decided to help you make diet changes, for example. Within a few weeks, you might see that your average has gone down 10 points, showing that you're making a significant impact on your health.

Note: You'll need to take a few minutes to read your meter's instruction booklet, in order to ensure that both the date and time are set correctly.

Sometimes the most important use of self-monitoring is to tell you if your BG is too low. Although the symptoms of low BG are often recognized (feeling sweaty, lightheaded, a fast heart rate, nervous, hungry), these symptoms are not exclusive to low BG. The same symptoms may be caused by extreme hunger or exercise (without a glucose low), or sometimes by feeling anxious or rushed. Checking your BG will tell you whether your symptoms need to be treated with carbohydrates because your BG is less than 70, or whether the symptoms are due to another cause.

If you are taking insulin as part of your diabetes treatment, checking your BG is pretty much essential. If you are taking a fast-acting insulin (such as Humalog, Novolog, Apidra, or regular insulin) then your glucose result before meals helps you choose the appropriate dose of "bolus" (mealtime) insulin you will need to cover the carbohydrates you will eat. If you are taking a long-lasting insulin (such as Lantus, NPH, or Levemir insulin), your morning BG readings can help you decide whether your daily "basal" (background) dose needs adjustment. If you find that your morning glucose readings are higher than you wish, checking your glucose before bed will provide you with additional vital information, such as how well you did at setting your short-acting doses during the day.

One of the primary purposes of long-lasting insulin is to keep your glucose from rising during the night. If your morning glucose is consistently more than 30 points higher than your bedtime glucose, you probably need an increase in your long-lasting insulin dose. If on the other hand, you find that your morning glucose is similar to your bedtime glucose, but that both of these results are higher than you wish, then your solution would be to take a higher dose of short-acting insulin at supper. This will bring your bedtime glucose down, allowing your long-acting insulin to keep your BG steady through the night.

Meanwhile, concerns about food are a major part of diabetes, and you need to learn how different foods affect your diabetes. Self-monitoring can help you do this. Perhaps you and your spouse differ over whether your supper choice was appropriate. The easiest way to solve this dilemma is to look at your BG before supper, and then again about three hours or more after eating. If these numbers are reasonable, then your supper choice was indeed reasonable in regard to your BG. (Remember that your food choices will also affect your lipid values and your blood pressure.)

Sometimes you may find that, in the morning, your BG is higher than you expected. This high morning reading can focus your attention on what you ate the previous evening. If it was a meal that contained more fat than usual such as pizza, this could bring your glucose up during the night because fat causes the carbohydrates to enter your blood stream more slowly. This means you might have had a reasonable reading before going to bed (you couldn't yet see the effects of the pizza). If this is the case, you can decide to choose pizza less often, or choose a smaller amount, or combine it with a walk after your meal.

It is also very helpful to check your BG before and after you exercise. Keep in mind that exercise has a stronger effect in decreasing insulin resistance than does any other intervention. In chapter 3, you developed a plan of action for your diabetes. If an increase in activity was part of your plan, self-monitoring will help you see the positive impact of exercise on your BG, and can provide information that you can use in planning the timing of your exercise. Remember that the major benefit of exercise is not the immediate effect that it has on lowering your BG, but rather the longer-term effect that it has on improving your insulin resistance. You will likely see a drop in your BG immediately following an exercise session, and the extent of this drop can help you gauge which activities give you the most benefit.

TRY IT WHEN YOU EXERCISE

NEXT TIME YOU'RE physically active for longer than twenty minutes, check to see what happens. No doubt you'll see a significant change.

BG: Before _____ After _____

The Best Times to Check Your BG

THE BEST TIMES to check your BG depend on your reasons for checking. If you are checking to choose your insulin doses, then the best times to check are before meals and at bedtime. Checking at the same times each day is helpful when your purpose is to assess improvement or change in your overall control.

If you do not need the information immediately to set insulin doses, then you needn't check every time period every day. Checking several times a week, but varying the times, should be sufficient. Just before a meal, and then three or four hours afterward, provides a useful timeframe for seeing the effects of that meal, while before and just after exercise will tell you the effects of that particular activity.

It's also important to use the little log book that comes with your meter to keep track of your numbers and look over them periodically. This is not just for your doctor, but for you. The numbers give you an immediate overview of your patterns, which will help you interpret the effects of your lifestyle changes and medications. That is, the data lets you see things like a tendency to run high in the afternoons (Are you eating too many carbs for lunch? Maybe you need a walk after eating.) or if you are too high nearly every morning (Time to adjust your dinner habits? Or maybe you need an overnight dose of insulin.). And of course, sharing your data with your medical providers allows them to better advise you as well. Instead of just giving you general one-size-fits-all recommendations that they may make to most other diabetes patients, they will be able to help you choose specific actions most appropriate for your own personal situation.

We are happy to report that BG monitoring has undergone a quiet revolution. Monitoring didn't become common until the 1980s. Even in the 1990s, glucose meters were often inaccurate and cumbersome to use, requiring larger drops of blood (more "ouch" to the stick) and taking almost a minute to deliver your result. Today's meters have made self-monitoring much easier, less painful, and much faster. Your personal glucose results will supply you with the regular feedback you need to keep your diabetes on track, along your road to success.

PART 2

Understanding Your Diabetes Tools

7 Moving Your Body
(a.k.a. Exercise)

Why Is Physical Activity So Important?

EXERCISE, PHYSICAL ACTIVITY, moving your body through space—whatever you want to call it—is perhaps the single most important action you can take in caring for your diabetes and for yourself. But before you start to groan about yet another addition to your busy life, or yet another burden you don't want to deal with, remember that you're already doing some exercise. Exercise is any planned physical activity that is in addition to your usual activities of daily living. And some people have jobs that entail a lot of physical activity: walking mail-delivery, construction work and farm work, bicycle messenger jobs, and so on. Also, if you care for a lively toddler, actively garden, or are a do-it-yourselfer home owner, you may be getting more exercise than you realize. Most of us, however, even if we have jobs that require some activity, are probably still not getting the amount of exercise that will best benefit our health. Instead, we humans now have stressful jobs that wear us out, but we don't use our muscles in the same way we did thousands of years ago.

Many people think about exercise in a narrow way, as in going to a gym or jogging for miles. But the physical activities that are good for your diabetes, as well as good for your heart, can come in a variety of forms, and it's very likely that you are already doing some of them. You can think about increasing your physical activity in three ways: extending or increasing the frequency of activities you're already doing; reintroducing activities that you enjoyed or successfully accomplished in the past; and adding in some new activities. Using some combination of these three approaches, your initial goal should be to 2.5 to 3 hours of added physical activity per week, at a moderate level. A moderate level of exercise is any activity that increases your heart rate, so that you can feel that you are making a little effort, but such that you are also comfortable enough to carry on a conversation. We discuss the level of exercise in more detail in the "How Much" section that follows.

What Kind of Activity Is Best?

THE BEST ACTIVITY for your diabetes, and for your heart, is **aerobic exercise**. This is basically any type of activity that moves your body through space, and increases your heart rate. Walking, dancing, bicycling, hiking, some types of gardening, and yard work are common aerobic activities. There are also two other forms of activity that are helpful in different ways:

Resistance training is using your muscles to push or pull against weighted objects, or anything that creates resistance. This could include light weights such as dumbbells, some types of calisthenics, or stretch resistance bands. Resistance training is helpful for building and maintaining muscle mass and strength, and for strengthening bones. When combined with aerobic exercise, it also has favorable effects on your glucose levels.

A third type of activity is **stretching**. Simple stretching exercises can improve your flexibility, and may serve as a helpful warm-up and cool-down for your aerobic exercise. Although stretching may not directly help your diabetes, it can improve your balance and flexibility and thus make it easier for you to perform your daily activities, and to participate in some more aerobic forms of exercise as well. There is some evidence that more formal stretching exercises like tai chi or yoga may be directly helpful to your diabetes, possibly helping to lower glucose and triglyceride levels. These activities can also be very helpful for improving mood, and decreasing stress, both of which are especially beneficial for people with diabetes.

Tell Me Why Again . . .

WHY IS EXERCISE the most important action for you to take when you have type 2 diabetes? Because exercise is the most potent treatment for insulin resistance (see chapter 13), which is one of the major causes contributing to your type 2 diabetes. Improvement in insulin resistance results from regular aerobic exercise, or a combination of aerobic exercise with some resistance training.

EXERCISE AS A DIABETES TREATMENT

THE DIABETES PREVENTION Program (DPP), a major research study completed in 2002, used a target of 2.5 hours a week of moderate physical activity such as brisk walking.

This amount of activity, which was within most people's reach, performed regularly over a four-year period, reduced the incidence of diabetes by over 55 percent.

The initial activity needs to be aerobic, but later you can add resistance training to your routine, up to equal amounts of time.

Most people with type 2 diabetes also find that exercise has an immediate effect on lowering their blood glucose—even aside from the improvement in insulin resistance. Checking your blood glucose before and after exercise can demonstrate this effect for you. If you find that your blood glucose is a little higher at one particular time of the day, then planning to exercise at that time might be helpful.

In fact, exercise can also add "dollars" your Diabetes Health Account in nearly every category, including beneficial effects on your lipids and blood pressure. Increasing your physical activity will decrease your LDL cholesterol, and is one of the more effective ways to increase your healthy HDL cholesterol. Just as for lowering your glucose, it's aerobic exercise that has the most benefit here.

You may have realized by now that improving your A1c, lowering your LDL cholesterol, increasing your HDL cholesterol, and lowering your blood pressure will all decrease your chances of cardiovascular disease. Since your heart is a muscle, aerobic exercise can improve your heart's strength, in a somewhat similar fashion to the way that lifting weights can make your biceps stronger. And a stronger heart means more funds in your Diabetes Health Account, toward a longer and healthier life. In addition to its beneficial effect on your heart muscle, exercise also has positive effects on your arteries that decrease the chance of atherosclerosis, which is the narrowing of arteries associated with heart disease, strokes, and peripheral vascular disease (disease of blood vessels outside the heart).

Feeling a little down about life and diabetes? Any type of exercise provides the additional benefit of improving your mood, helping to combat the frustrations that we all experience to some degree. This is because exercise stimulates your brain to release hormones called *endorphins*, which work to suppress sensations of pain and produce a sense of well-being. Exercise also increases levels of *serotonin*, a substance proven to stave off depression and aggressive behavior. And last, not least: exercise can help control your weight, and is one the necessary components for any long-term success with weight loss.

Exercise and Weight Loss

ON THE SUBJECT of fitness, many people, especially with diabetes, are concerned about losing weight. This is problematic for two reasons: first, the effects of weight on your health are much less influential than you might think; and secondly, losing weight is known to be difficult.

Although newspapers and magazines are full of warnings about weight gain and the nation's obesity epidemic, these articles generally have a misleading overemphasis on food and diet, while ignoring the effects of sedentary lifestyle. That is, when weight and fitness are considered together, the effect of fitness on your health trumps weight. We know this from clinical evidence: there is clear proof that Americans, especially young people, are increasingly less active. There is also clear proof that this decrease in activity, and the resulting decrease in overall fitness, are related to a number of health problems, including diabetes and heart disease. People at the lower end of the fitness spectrum can have up to five times greater risk of heart problems than those who are physically active regularly. In fact, clinical research shows that a moderate level of physical activity (several hours a week) can decrease the risk of a heart attack by over 50 percent.

Of course, this national trend of decreasing physical activity is associated with an increase in weight. However, the effect of weight alone on your health—except at the extremes of thinness and obesity—is actually minimal.

Another worrisome health trend is the increasing consumption of calorie-rich convenience foods and beverages, including fast foods, sports drinks, and non-diet soft drinks that all add calories but lack any health benefits. These processed foods and beverages contain the kind of fats that increase your LDL, instead of the heart-healthy fats that decrease it, and they lack the healthful fiber and nutrients that fruit and vegetables provide.

This trend in food choices is also associated with weight gain, of course, but keep in mind that it's the poor food choices, and not your weight itself, that cause the direct damage to your health. In fact, studies have shown that when people make healthy changes in their food consumption, they improve their improve glucose metabolism (BG levels)—even if they don't lose weight in the process. Again, the makeup of the food you eat is more important to your overall health than its direct effect on your weight.

The message here is actually a simple one: increasing your physical activity and making healthy food choices have the major effects on your health, which is more important than the number you get when you step on a scale. Furthermore, if losing weight remains one of your goals, then the path to follow is twofold: increasing your physical activity and making healthy food choices.

REAL PEOPLE:
EXERCISE IS NOT JUST FOR WEIGHT LOSS

LORETTA, A KINDLY grandmother from the Deep South, was diagnosed with type 2 diabetes in her mid-sixties. She was substantially overweight, and decided right away to start an exercise routine in order to shed up to sixty unwanted pounds.

Luckily, she found a class at a local clinic that fit her tastes: a personal coach helping a group of people in a small gym that had a treadmill and several stationary bikes, which were particularly good for the problem hip that often bothered Loretta. She quickly made friends with four other ladies there, and they continued to exercise together even after the class ended.

Loretta was delighted to see that within the first two months, she'd lost ten pounds. But then things leveled off. She continued to exercise three to four times a week, but as the months melted into years, no additional weight loss occurred. You can imagine her frustration.

Yet when her doctor asked her how she felt, she had to admit, she'd never had more energy. She found that she was able to maneuver better in the grocery store, bending and pushing her cart with ease. And she could now take long walks with her granddaughter, which would have been unthinkable before.

> **Loretta's A1c result also dropped from 7.8 to under 6.5, and has stayed there for the last five years. In short, the exercise has made her a much healthier person, even though she still isn't thin.**
>
> The health impact of exercise goes far beyond weight loss; a fit overweight person is much healthier than an unfit overweight person.

The benefits of exercise are amazing in their breadth: improving insulin resistance, lowering blood glucose, increasing HDL cholesterol, lowering LDL cholesterol, improving blood pressure, strengthening your heart, helping your mood, and assisting with weight loss. Does exercise seem too familiar or mundane to have all these wonderful effects? Well, think again. Human bodies were built for physical activity; it is part of the natural system that keeps our bodies healthy. If there were a pill or a surgical procedure that produced these great benefits of exercise, without side effects, everyone in the world would be taking it or doing it. But there is no legitimate artificial substitute for exercise yet, and there's also no way you can deny its central importance in improving your health—even if you didn't have diabetes.

How Much Is Enough?

THE AMOUNT OF exercise you need in order to obtain the benefits is probably less than you think. In the Diabetes Prevention Program mentioned above, participants averaged about 2 to 3 hours of brisk walking per week. To maximize the benefits of exercise, it helps to spread out your activity through the week, so that you are doing some type of physical activity at least four days a week. Since our busy days can make long sessions difficult, try breaking up your exercise during the day to make it easier to fit into your schedule. Two fifteen-minute sessions can be just as helpful as one thirty-minute session.

There are several ways to gauge your exercise. Frequency and duration determine the total time spent on exercise, while intensity of the exercise is also important. Intensity can be measured by calories burned per minute, watts, or **metabolic equivalents (METs)**—all unit measures of intensity than can often be displayed on treadmills, elliptical machines, or other gym equipment. Although the term may be least familiar to you, METs are actually the preferred measurement for exercise physiologists. One MET is the amount of energy that you expend when your body is at rest (about 1 kilocalorie per kilogram per hour, for the numerically inclined).

Mild activity such as slow walking is about 2.5 METs, meaning that you expend about two and a half times as much energy when you walk slowly, as when you sit still. When it comes to exercise, mild forms of activity are better than doing nothing, but are mostly helpful for transitioning you to higher levels of activity. An initial goal should be to perform "moderate activity," at a level of 3 to 6 METs.

Below are some common activities grouped by effort. These are just approximations, because the energy and effort required vary by person, age, fitness level, environment, and other factors.

Light Activity (less than 3 METs)
- Walking (less than 3 mph, or more than 20 minutes to walk a mile)
- Shopping
- Stretching, yoga
- Child care
- Sitting in whirlpool
- Arguing (even with hand waving)
- Playing a musical instrument
- Driving

- Bird watching
- Talking on phone
- Classroom instruction
- Fishing
- Light housework
- Cooking

Moderate Activity (between 3 and 6 METs)
- Walking (3 mph or faster)
- Dancing
- Riding a bicycle
- Riding a stationary bicycle, with light effort
- Swimming (moderate pace)
- Low-impact aerobics
- Vacuuming
- Moderate housework
- Mowing the lawn
- Gardening
- Golf
- Kayaking
- Water aerobics
- Softball

Vigorous Activity (greater than 6 METs)
- Jogging, running
- Bicycling (faster than 10 mph)
- Backpacking
- Racquetball
- Tennis
- Soccer
- Swimming (sprinting or long-distance)
- Basketball
- Rollerblading
- Rope jumping
- Canoeing

- Skiing
- Snow-shoeing

A more comprehensive list of METs associated with specific activities is available from the University of South Carolina, compiled by Dr. Barbara Ainsworth, at http://prevention.sph.sc.edu/tools/docs/documents_compendium.pdf.

In terms of intensity, you get the most benefit from moving your muscles as you start, not *overworking* them. To check yourself, take the **Talk Test** while you're exercising: can you hold a conversation, or are you huffing and puffing too hard to speak? If the latter is the case, you're overdoing it. Also, you can do multiple short sessions of exercise throughout the day, rather than pushing too hard or trying to block in a longer, single session. In fact, frequency is important; you'll get more out of several short sessions per week than you would out of just one or two long sessions.

Thoughts on Your Own Exercise Plan

WHEN YOU THINK about your own exercise plan, remember the approach we discussed earlier in the chapter. Look for ways to add exercise by extending activities that you are already doing. If you are walking part of the way to work each day, could you extend the distance? If you're going to the gym twice a week, could you add in a third visit? Were there times in the past when you exercised more often, and enjoyed it? What was your routine then, and can you blend a little of that into your current plan? Take another look at the list of moderate activities, and see if there is something that you would enjoy adding. Perhaps splitting your exercise plan among several different things that suit your lifestyle, such briskly walking for twenty minutes during your lunch hour on workdays, and bike riding with your family on weekends.

REAL PEOPLE:
SAVING YOUR EYES BY MOVING YOUR BODY

JUDITH WAS TWENTY-SIX years old and had type 1 diabetes since age seven when her eye doctor suddenly discovered something "cloudy" at the back of her eye during an annual exam. Judith had always taken good care of herself, and consistently taken her medications. So she was especially shocked and frightened.

It turned out to be the beginnings of a dreaded "cotton-wool spot," a grayish-white or yellowish patch of discoloration in the nerve fiber layer of the eye, which indicates swelling there. This swelling is almost always due to reduced blood flow through the retinal vessels, and is typically an early indication of diabetic eye disease, common in both type 1 and type 2 diabetes.

What did the doctor prescribe? To her surprise, he recommended cardio exercise (raising her heart rate for at least thirty minutes at a stretch) three times a week—"and come back to see me in a few months." That was in May.

Judith took to the gym, consistently. Nothing Olympic, but very regular and with gradually increasing intensity. She also went to see her endocrinologist, who determined that her blood pressure was too high as well. He prescribed a daily dose of 2.5mg of Altace, an ACE inhibitor designed to reduce the risk of heart disease (by contracting muscles around blood vessels, thus increasing blood flow).

Judith took the pills, of course, and she kept at her gym efforts. She checked her glucose levels religiously, so she could intervene immediately when she was too high.

By August, with her new regime of regular exercise, the verdict was overturned. Her eye had cleared up in just a few months, and she's now complication free—and in great shape to boot. No one's ever been happier not to have skipped that

> annual eye exam. And no one's ever appreciated the value of
> exercise more.
>
> "Small health miracles" can be easily accomplished just by
> committing to some kind of regular exercise routine.

Don't Go Too Low

What about exercise and your blood glucose? Will your blood
glucose go too low, below 70 (a condition called hypoglycemia),
when you exercise? First off, be aware that if you are *not* taking the
specific diabetes medications below, you will not need to snack, or
even worry about blood glucose lows. If you *are* taking insulin, or
one of the medications listed in the following table, then it will be
useful for you to carry your meter and check your blood glucose
before, after, and possibly during exercise.

DIABETES MEDICATIONS AND
RISK OF HYPOGLYCEMIA

NOT AT RISK	AT RISK
Glucophage (Metformin)	**Insulin** (all types)
Avandia (Rosiglitizone)	**Diabeta, Micronase, Glynase, Glucovance** (contains Glyburide)
Avandamet (Metformin/ Rosiglitizone)	**Glucotrol, Glucotrol XL, Metaglip** (contains Glipizide)
Actos (Pioglitazone)	**Amaryl** (Glimepiride)
Precose (Acarbose)	**Prandin** (Repaglinide)
Glyset (Miglitol)	**Starlix** (Natelinide)

If you're taking any of the pills in the right-hand column, then you'll
want to be sure your blood glucose is above 100 mg/dL before start-

ing exercise. You should also carry some form of fast-acting carbohy-drate with you at all times to treat lows if they occur. About 15 grams of carbohydrate should do the trick. This could be glucose tablets, a few pieces of hard candy (not chocolate), or a sugar-containing drink.

If you are taking any of the listed medicines and find that your blood glucose is under 90 mg/dL at *the end* of your activity sessions, then you may need a small snack of about 15 grams of carbohydrate while you're active, to prevent going too low. This could be a hand-ful of crackers, a small piece of fruit, or a handful of raisins.

The most common strategy for insulin users is to reduce the dose of insulin at the meal prior to exercise. It's wise to keep a log of insulin doses, time of workout, activity, and what happened, so you can make a plan to treat your own pattern. Your doctor or dia-betes educator can help you here.

Note that diabetes is *not* a barrier to intense exercise—even at the Olympic level—as long as you have the patience to learn how to adjust your medications and food intake appropriately.

In most cases, you won't need to take an extra snack for your exercise. Walking two miles burns only about 180 calories, which is not that much, so you don't need to include a 200-calorie snack along with your walk.

Working Around Medical Conditions

If you are over forty, or have specific health concerns (other than the diabetes) that might be affected by increasing your exercise, it makes sense to talk with your doctor before starting new activities. This is especially true if you have symptoms of chest discomfort or tightness, shortness of breath, or pain in your neck or your arm when you exercise, or if you have a history of high blood pressure or heart disease. These medical concerns do not mean that you shouldn't exercise—to the contrary, we know that exercise is very helpful in improving these medical conditions. It just means that you will benefit from a little extra advice from your health-care team. They may want to perform a routine exercise tolerance test (a treadmill test), or give you some specific recommendations to follow when you are first starting your exercise.

Don't Stop Now: Maintaining Momentum

Starting exercise is one thing, but maintaining it over the long term is quite another. Why doesn't everyone exercise regularly, since it has such a major impact on health, and can elevate one's mood? There are lots of reasons not to exercise, of course. But if you don't find a way around these excuses, you will be missing one of the most important tools for building up your health.

The most common barrier is not having enough time. We all lead busy lives; work, travel time, and family responsibilities can seem to fill our days and weeks completely. So how do you add exercise? Combining it with regular errands or routines can be helpful. Walking a little further for your morning coffee or paper, parking a mile away from work or at the other end of the lot from the stores you customarily drive right up to at the mall, or using your bike for running errands instead of public transportation or driving are ways to add in bits of extra activity during the day. You are the one who best knows your daily schedule and responsibilities: What would be the easiest time to slot in your exercise? Maybe it would be easier to slot in two shorter exercise sessions. If inclement weather puts a damper on an outdoor activity, try substituting a different indoor one instead of going totally AWOL on your regimen until the seasons change.

Perhaps you know that exercise is important, but each day new demands on your time seem to pop up, and each of these new demands pushes off the exercise to a later time, until finally you run out of time. If this happens frequently, take a moment to reevaluate the priorities of your day. If you really *know* that exercise will bring you many positive benefits, perhaps something this important needs a regular "appointment time." If you schedule your exercise as if it were any other non-negotiable responsibility, you'll make more of an effort to plan other demands around this vital commitment, rather than moving or missing your exercise in favor of less essential activities.

Another common barrier is simply finding exercise unenjoyable or boring. This is especially common when other people, like your health-care provider or your spouse, are the ones urging you to exercise. Think about *your* reasons for wanting to exercise, and consider the priority that *you* wish to give to your exercise. Maybe you could try a new type of activity that might be more fun, such as square, line, or ballroom dancing, which combines movement with music and socializing. Consider less traditional forms of exercise such as introductory martial arts or tai chi, or perhaps outdoor hiking or orienteering (scouting unfamiliar territory with a group of hikers).

Joining an organized exercise program, so that you are not doing it alone, may also be helpful. Lots of shopping malls now offer morning "mall-walking" programs, local YMCA's often have surprisingly nice facilities at low prices, or your local hospital may offer fitness programs that can get you started in a supervised way. With so many people prioritizing exercise these days, you can likely find a partner to join you: a coworker who's interested in walking at lunchtime, or a neighbor or family member who can join you in the morning or evening. For many people, having company makes exercise much easier, and adds a social aspect to your health improvement as well. And don't forget the simple strategy of integrating exercise into your daily routine, such as riding your bike or walking to work on a regular basis. This can be very enjoyable, and a good way to fit regular activity into your established routine.

Stress or physical discomfort can turn you off from exercise, too. Many of us are increasingly stressed by our work and personal lives, and this stress can produce a fatigue that makes exercising seem an unlikely option—just something that would make you feel even more tired. But exercise actually creates a sense of renewed energy. Once you begin some regular exercise, you'll soon find that it supplies you with a little extra energy, as your body tunes itself to a healthier metabolism.

If you have back or knee pain, or arthritis, and fear that exercise will cause you more discomfort, start slowly. Spread your exercise throughout the day, in multiple ten-minute sessions. Begin by choosing activities that may cause less discomfort, such as cycling, swimming, or armchair exercises for a gentle start. Although chronic pain can make it harder to get started, we know that steady persistence will end up helping to ease it, as the muscles around your joints become stronger and can offer more support. If you are bothered by arthritis or specific joints, your health-care provider or a physical therapist can help you include specific exercises that will stretch and strengthen the appropriate muscles.

If you've been inactive for a long time, you may feel that you are too out of shape, or too overweight to exercise. Again, begin by spreading your exercise throughout the day, and starting with some easier activities, which will get you moving down the road toward increased activity.

THREE TRUTHS ABOUT EXERCISE

1. Exercise is the most effective and portable stress-management tool on the market.
2. Health-wise, being physically fit is much more important than being thin.
3. If there's ever been a case where something is better than nothing, it's moving your body.

We cannot overemphasize the importance of being physically active. This is because nothing goes further towards staving off diabetic complications. And regular exercise can make you feel surprisingly good: it gives you more energy, helps reduce stress, eases tension and anxiety, and improves sleep, and even improves your sex life, according to clinical studies. Exercise makes you feel better about yourself, your quality of life, and your independence as a person with diabetes.

8 Dealing with Food

FOOD + DIET = TWO of the most charged words associated with diabetes. This is the area that most frustrates and worries people with diabetes, and the area most often associated with exasperating input like, "Can you eat that?" and "No sweets, no bread, no pasta!" (Which for many people translates into "No life!")

Diet recommendations seem to come at you from all directions: from health-care providers, TV, newspapers, magazines, and the Internet (including e-mail spam, which offers advice generally as healthful as real Spam). Low-fat, low-carb, South Beach, Zone, Pritikin, Atkins, and many other diets are hyped continually, not to mention the grassroots spread of odd single-food diets such as the Grapefruit Diet and the Cabbage Soup Diet. (The fact that you yourself haven't written a diet book seems to put you in the minority.)

Despite this barrage of restrictive suggestions, we'd like to clarify that there is no such thing as a food that a person with diabetes can *never* eat. Even sweets, chocolate, and other favorites are possible. But you will need some information about the nutritional content of the foods you eat, combined with your knowledge of your own specific A1c, lipids, and blood pressure, to keep your health in check.

> **WHILE THE GOOD** news is that you can eat anything, it is also true that you can't eat everything—at least not all at once.

We believe that a good deal of the confusion and frustration around food comes from recommendations that are too general—assuming that a single healthy diet is the same for everyone. In fact, there are many quite varied diets that can be called healthy, and, more important, each person should be tailoring what is healthy to his or her own specific health needs. Do you know your own specific needs? For patients with diabetes, there are four general aspects to consider when thinking about your nutrition plan:

- Your glucose control, that is, your A1c
- Your lipid levels
- Your blood pressure
- Your weight

Each of these requires a different focus: carbohydrates for your A1c; fats for your lipid levels; salt, fruits, and vegetables for your blood pressure; and attention to calories and perhaps carbohydrate content for controlling your weight.

We have found that almost everyone eats a fair amount of healthy foods already. The problems lie more in (1) choosing the foods that address your own body's specific needs, and (2) establishing portion control. Therefore, most people don't need to change their diet drastically, which is good news, since drastic diet changes rarely last. Instead, you need to think of *modifying* your diet: building on the good parts, while limiting the less helpful parts. To do this, you'll need to learn more about the contents of the food you already eat.

What's in Food, Anyway?

ALL FOOD IS made up of three parts: carbohydrate, fat, and protein (see the "Basic Elements" below). Some foods, such as fruit, bread, chicken, or olive oil, consist mainly of only one of these elements. Other foods, such as beans, contain a combination of these elements. Our meals typically contain combinations of all three. The amount of carbohydrate, protein, and fat in your food directly correlates with its number of calories: there are 4 calories for every gram of carbohydrate and protein, and 7 calories for every gram of fat.

Fiber content and calorie density are also important elements to consider when making your food choices.

THE BASIC ELEMENTS OF FOOD

- **CARBOHYDRATE** = the sugars and starches found in grains, fruits, vegetables, and dairy products.

  This category includes all obviously sugary foods like sweets, fruit, and sugar itself, along with grains and starchy foods (pasta, potatoes, rice) that break down to glucose in your body. Carbs usually make up the bulk of your diet, and are used by your body for basic energy needs.
- **PROTEIN** = the major component in meats, such as beef, pork, chicken, and fish. Protein is also present in some vegetables and in legumes, such as beans.

  You need protein to build and repair body tissue. Protein can also provide energy for your body if carbs are not available for fuel. Your muscles, organs, bones, skin, and many of the hormones in your body are made from protein.
- **FAT** = the densest form of calories, present in pure form in oils, necessary for frying (the reason potato chips are so high in fat), and also present to varying degrees in meats, dairy products, and nuts (along with protein).

> Three types of fat are found in food: saturated, unsaturated, and trans fat. Your body does need fat, but in very limited quantities—and never in the form of trans fat.

How to Read Food Labels

Learning the makeup of your present diet is essential, and probably means acquiring a few new skills. One important skill is how to make sense of food labels. Nowadays, food producers are required to list both the ingredients and the nutritional value of their products on a detailed label. This is good news for you, because the label provides you with everything you need to know about the food (except for how it tastes). Let's walk through a typical label, pictured below.

Serving size

The first thing to do is to look closely at the *serving size*. We cannot emphasize this enough.

This is crucial because the estimated serving size is often not the amount of food you will actually eat. And the other numbers on the label will be meaningless unless they reflect your actual serving size.

For example, the label shown here is from a 4½-ounce bag of potato chips. It provides information about the serving size in two ways, which can be very confusing. First, it gives the serving by the number of chips (useful for the many people who routinely count their individual potato chips before eating them). Then it gives the number of servings per bag: five. We know that the most people buying this size bag of chips are not thinking of sharing it with four friends. An entire bag is 750 calories and that many chips contain a whopping 75 percent of your daily recommended fat intake. So be aware that many small or individual-seeming packages of snack foods actually contain multiple servings, and adjust your consumption of them accordingly.

```
Nutrition Facts
Serving Size  11
Servings Per Container  5
```

Amount Per Serving	%Daily Value*
Calories 150	
Total Fat 10g	4%
Saturated Fat 2.5g	0%
Cholesterol 0mg	0%
Sodium 180mg	5%
Total Carbohydrate 15g	10%
Dietary Fiber 2g	
Sugars 0g	0%
Other Carbohydrate 0g	0%
Protein 2g	
Vitamin A	10%
Vitamin C	10%
Calicum	0%
Iron	0%

* Percent Daily Values are based on a 2,000 calorie diet. Your daily values may be higher or lower depending on your calorie needs:

	Calories:	2,000	2,500
Total Fat	Less than	65g	80g
Sat Fat	Less than	20g	25g
Cholesterol	Less than	300mg	300mg
Sodium	Less than	3,2400mg	
2,400mg			
Total Carbohydrate		300g	375g
Dietary Fiber		25g	30g

Calories per gram:
Fat 9 • Carbohydrate 4 • Protein 4

Ingredients: Potatoes, Vegetable Oil (Contains One or More of the Following: Corn, Cottonseed, or Sunflower Oil), and Salt.

Total calories

Next on the label is the total number of calories, in this case 150 *per serving* (750 divided by 5 servings). Remember that this is the number of calories in *one serving*, not in the whole bag! The label also shows the total number of calories per serving that come from fat: 90 calories. Since 90 is more than half of the 150 total calories, this means you are getting more calories from the fat used to fry the chips than from the other two food components of the actual potatoes, protein and carbohydrate, combined.

Percentages

Listed to the right of each individual food component is a *percent of daily value*. This information is based on the USDA's recommendations for healthy amounts of carbs, protein, sodium, fat, and so on, which you should eat each day. The percentage shows how much of each component you get in a single serving of this food, compared with the recommended daily values. For example, one serving of these chips provides 10 percent of the total amount of vitamin C that you should eat in a day.

Fats: the Good, the Bad, and the Ugly

Next on the label come *fats*, important because of their high calorie content, and their effect on cardiovascular disease. What's important to know is that the *total fat content* is not enough information for you. It does help you determine how calorie-packed the food is, but you need to know more about the specific makeup of the fats to determine how healthy they are for your heart. The three main types of fats are: mono and polyunsaturated fats, saturated fats, and trans fats—which you can think of, respectively, as "the good, the bad, and the ugly."

Always look first at the amount of bad and ugly fats on a food label, since these can have a significant negative impact on your health. Saturated fats increase your LDL cholesterol, and trans fats have an even worse effect on your cholesterol and your risk of heart disease. Saturated fats are found in meats, particularly beef, as well as in dairy products. These unhealthy fats are present in even higher amounts in palm and coconut oil.

Trans fats do not occur naturally, and are therefore found in processed foods, and fast foods such as french fries. These fats were not specifically listed on food labels until 2006. Now that labeling is required for trans fats, and consumers have become very alerted to their unhealthiness, they are starting to disappear, as food manufacturers make adjustments. However, many convenience, snack, and fast foods continue to contain them.

Now, the good fats—poly- and monounsaturated—can actually decrease your LDL cholesterol, increase your healthy HDL cholesterol, and decrease your chance of heart disease. They still pack the same calorie content, but substituting poly- and monounsaturated fats for the saturated and trans fats in your diet can have a very healthy outcome. The concentration of these healthy fats is higher in chicken and turkey than in beef and pork, and fish contain some of the healthiest fats of all. Oils such as canola, olive, and soybean also contain very healthy mixtures of fats. So the point is not to eliminate fats from your diet, but to choose only the healthiest kinds, in moderation, because they actually clean your blood vessels of LDL cholesterol.

Overall, experts recommend that fats should make up not more than 30 to 35 percent of your overall daily calorie intake. This means that if you were following a 2,000-calorie meal plan, you should be eating no more than 60 to 70 grams of fat per day mostly monounsaturated sources. Again, avoid trans fats, which sabotage these good fats' ability to keep you healthy.

Cholesterol

After fats, you will see *cholesterol* listed on the food label. Foods that are higher in cholesterol are the same ones that are high in saturated fats: generally meat and dairy, plus eggs. Here's the interesting thing, though: while your body's cholesterol levels are of major importance to your health, the cholesterol content of the food you eat has only a minor impact on your cholesterol levels. Most of the cholesterol in your blood is made by your liver, fueled by the types of fat that you eat. Therefore the amount and type of fats that you eat have a bigger health impact than does the cholesterol you consume. Nevertheless, current FDA recommendations are to eat no more than 300 mg/day of cholesterol.

Sodium

Next, you will see *sodium* listed. Sodium is the important component of salt (sodium chloride) that's in your salt shaker, but it is also present, sometimes in surprising amounts, in prepared foods, especially in baked goods that use baking powder or baking soda as leavening agents. Yet even high-sodium foods may not taste overtly salty. You're better off skipping prepared foods that contain hidden sources of sodium, and instead preparing food fresh and adding the salt yourself if desired. You should be able to get the flavor you want with a lesser amount of sodium than food manufacturers typically use—or perhaps forgo it in part or completely with the substitution of herbs and spices. Current FDA recommendations are about a teaspoon of sodium a day (about 2,300 mg)—less, if you have high blood pressure that's sensitive to your salt intake.

Carbohydrates

Carbohydrates come next on the label. These are the most important foods you eat, comprising the main source of energy for your body. As a person with diabetes, you will want to look closely at the carb content of foods, which has a direct impact on raising your BG levels. We've devoted a separate section in this chapter (page 128) to carbohydrates. But for the moment, let's finish reading that nutrition label.

Fiber

Fiber is actually another type of carbohydrate, although it does not raise your BG levels and actually has some pretty amazing health effects. Fiber is the structural portion of fruits, vegetables, grains, nuts, and legumes that cannot be digested or absorbed by your body. Therefore, fiber does not provide calories. Some fibers add bulk to your meals, helping you feel full, whereas others have a laxative effect on your digestive system. Fiber comes primarily from wheat, corn, or oat bran; legumes (cooked dried beans and peas); nuts; and vegetables and fruit, especially when raw.

Very large amounts of fiber (approximately 50 grams per day) have been shown to improve BG levels, lipids, and even insulin levels in the body. Also, a diet high in fiber and whole grains has been shown to slightly reduce risk of heart disease and may reduce the chance of some types of cancer, improve digestive health, and help with weight control.

Fiber and whole grains go hand in hand. Whole grains include all three parts of a grain—the bran, germ, and endosperm. The fiber, vitamins, minerals, and hundreds of **phytonutrients** (the health-protective substances in plant foods) found in grains work together against heart disease and may help with glucose control. So look for foods that list whole-grain ingredients first, for example: whole-wheat flour, whole oats, whole-grain corn, or brown rice, because an ingredients list always starts with the item of greatest volume within the food (see details under "Ingredients" on page 126). And try to eat vegetables raw or lightly cooked, rather than peeled and cooked to a pulp, to maximize their fiber. For example, if you usually eat only the florets and discard the thick stems of broccoli, try slicing the stalks thinly into "coins" and quickly stir-frying them, for a tasty boost of fiber.

No matter how you slice it, lots of fiber is good for you. Experts recommend at least 20 to 35 grams per day, or even up to 50 grams per day if you have type 2 diabetes and need to lose weight. But if you're not used to eating fiber, increase your intake gradually, to give your digestive system time to adjust—otherwise you may feel quite gassy and experience cramps at the start.

Protein

You need *protein* to build and repair body tissue. Protein can also provide energy for your body if carbs are not available for fuel. Your muscles, organs, bones, skin, and many of the hormones in your body are made from protein.

Meat, poultry, and fish are good sources of protein. Milk, yogurt, and beans are examples of foods that contain both carbohydrate and protein. Any food containing at least 5 grams of protein per serving is considered a good source of it.

Most adults need about two servings per day of 3 to 4 ounces of protein, depending on your weight goals and overall health. Remember that many of your protein sources also contain fat, so you should choose foods with this in mind.

Ingredients

At the very bottom of the food label, you will find the food's *ingredients* listed in descending order by weight. This means the food contains the highest amount of the first items listed, and less of each item as you read down the list. This part of the label also provides more detailed information about the specific types of fats the food contains. As noted earlier, avoid eating anything that lists "partially hydrogenated" fats or oils (= trans fats) as a component.

Also, you will frequently find listed corn syrup, and sometimes high-dextrose corn syrup, and dextrose added to prepared and processed foods, often in foods you don't even think of as requiring a sweetener. You may be surprised to see, for example, that one of the main ingredients of hot dogs is corn syrup or dextrose. Manufactured breads often contain it, too. Why? Corn syrup is rich in carbohydrates, and dextrose is another scientific name for glucose, or sugar. Most people do not buy cranberry juice cocktail with the purpose of drinking high-fructose corn syrup, yet it is the third chief ingredient after water and cranberries. Good news: you do not have to give up eating processed foods entirely. More and more tasty alternative products can be found at your supermarket, and at health food stores. But always read the ingredients list, not just the large labels on the front of the package, to be sure.

ADDITIONAL FOOD LABEL LINGO

SUGAR-FREE	Less than 0.5 gram of sugar per serving
NO SUGAR ADDED	No sugar added during processing
FAT-FREE	Less than 0.5 grams of fat per serving
LOW-FAT	3 grams fat or less per serving
LOW SATURATED FAT	1 gram or less of saturated fat per serving
LOW CHOLESTEROL	20 mg or less of any kind of fat, and 2 grams or less of saturated fat per serving
LOW-SODIUM	140 milligrams or less of sodium per serving
LOW-CALORIE	40 calories or less per serving
LEAN	Less than 10 grams of fat, 4 grams of saturated fat, and 95 mg of cholesterol per serving
LIGHT	One-third fewer calories or one-half less fat than the regular version; or no more than half the sodium of the regular version
REDUCED	25% less of a specific nutrient, or 25% fewer calories than the regular version

What about foods without labels? Foods that don't come in cans or packages are very often good choices, but how can you discover their nutrition information? If you like going online, a great source is www.nal.usda.gov/fnic/foodcomp/search/. This Web site allows you to search for the nutritional content of almost any food, and is considered a definitive source for most information about food content. You can also buy a guide to food content. See the titles listed at the end of the next section, for a start.

All about Carbohydrates

DESPITE ALL THE fanfare around low-carb and no-carb foods, carbohydrates are the most important foods you eat, comprising the main source of energy for your body. Sugars, such as glucose, are the simplest forms of carbohydrate, and almost all carbohydrate can be converted to glucose by your body. Glucose is the common fuel used by your cells. If you don't eat enough carbohydrate to supply this glucose directly, your body will be starving for energy; it will release glucose from stores in the liver and muscle tissue, or form glucose from noncarbohydrate sources in a process called *ketosis*. So keep in mind that even though carbohydrates have a bigger impact on your BG levels than fats or protein, they are not to be avoided. Remember, they are your essential source of energy. Nevertheless, you do need to be aware of the carbohydrate content of your food, especially if your A1c is not in your target range, because limiting carbohydrates can be a useful tool for regulating your A1c.

Carbohydrate is present in vegetables, fruits, bread, pasta, and other foods made from grains and dairy products. Sugars such as table sugar (sucrose) and glucose are also carbohydrates, and are listed separately on food labels. Despite their separate listing, they have the same effect on your nutrition and BG as do most carbohydrates. Potatoes, white bread, juice, and most desserts and snacks, be they sweet or savory, all have similar effects on BG. What this means in practical terms is that there's no reason for you to avoid sugars altogether; rather, you need to have a balanced amount of carbohydrates in your diet.

CARB FACTS

- **A CARB IS A CARB**—most carbs, whatever kind they are, have the same effect on your body. Be they sugars or starches, they all convert to glucose in the end.
- **SUGAR-FREE IS NOT CARB-FREE**—don't let marketing labels fool you into believing that some carbs "don't count." Such products may still contain significant amounts of starches or alternative sweeteners, such as honey or maple syrup, that still convert to glucose.
- **FIBER DOES THE TRICK**—a high fiber content in a food (more than 5 grams per serving) can reduce the impact of that food on your BG, by moving it quickly out of your body before its carbs can be fully absorbed.

The Glycemic Index: Fast- and Slow-Acting Carbs

While it is true that most of our commonly eaten carbohydrates have similar effects on your BG, some carbohydrates do have advantages over others. These advantages stem from containing fiber and other nutrients present in foods such as fruits and vegetables. These extra-beneficial carbohydrates tend to be in the group of foods with a so-called low glycemic index.

The **glycemic index (GI)** is an attempt to scientifically determine the impact of individual foods on your BG levels. To set the GI value of a particular food, say a slice of bread, ten volunteers eat 50 grams (about 2 ounces) of the bread in the morning after fasting, and their BG is measured over the next two hours. The total rise in glucose during this two-hour time period is calculated. Several days later, the same ten volunteers drink 50 grams of glucose, and have their BG measured in the same way over the next two hours. Then the two glucose sums are compared, and the difference in value between the test food and the ingested glucose becomes the GI value for the tested food.

You can find the GI value of hundreds of foods in a database maintained by the University of Sydney, Australia, at www.glycemic index.com. You can even submit samples of a food, along with a check, and the research team will measure its GI for you.

Foods with lower GI values have a lesser impact on BG in the first two hours after you've eaten them. These foods need longer to absorb into your system. For this reason, lower GI foods could be good choices for people with diabetes. (Low-GI carbohydrate foods are otherwise known as *slow-acting carbs*.)

Yet, as easy as it sounds, the glycemic index can becomes a little complicated when you're trying to apply it in real life. Foods don't always affect your BG the way you would expect them to, based on their GI value, due to a number of variables: most of your food is not eaten directly after fasting, as it was during the GI testing; and also you eat foods in various combinations and amounts, not the single, precise quantities used in the tests. Their method of cooking and even their age (think ripe versus overripe bananas) also changes foods' GI impact. In the final analysis, however, using the glycemic index *or* relying on the recommendation to eat more fiber, fruits, and vegetables, will both lead you in the same general direction.

Keep in mind that whole, unprocessed foods, and meals prepared from scratch, will always be better for you than any fabricated low-carb product. Manufactured diet foods are often extremely high in fat and chemicals, and has in some cases even been altered specifically to be indigestible, so that your so-called "free" chocolate will create a nasty stomachache. Also, all too often, a prepared food that leaves out one element will overcompensate with another, so that the product will still taste good. Thus a low-carb bread might be loaded with salt or fats or artifical ingredients you really don't want in your body. We can't stress enough to read the nutrition and ingredient labels of *all* manufactured food products, even when they are advertised as being healthy.

Know Your Carbs

Carbohydrates are central to most diets. As we've just discussed, they provide your most essential source of energy, and since they have the major impact on your BG, it's important to know the *total carb content* of your food, rather than just the sugar content. It makes good sense to spread out your carb intake throughout the day, both to provide a more steady source of fuel, and to avoid large quantities of carbs hitting your diabetic metabolism all at once (which will make your BG shoot up).

Message in a Bottle

What you drink also counts. Since most of us are *not* trying to gain weight, it's useful to avoid forms of sugar that skirt around being listed literally as sugar. These are often found in nondiet beverages that are sweetened with corn products or fruit juices, or "natural" sweeteners such as honey, molasses, malt, and maple syrup. Soy and nut milks usually contain sweeteners too. Of course it's important to drink liquids when you're thirsty, but unless you are both thirsty and trying to gain weight, you won't need the added carbs and calories of most soft and sports drinks—and these include the trendy waters (still and spritzers) and teas that contain juices or other sweeteners as flavoring agents. Always read the ingredients list of bottled beverages to check for carbs.

USE YOUR FISTS

CARB COUNTING is a tool for managing your BG levels by calculating the precise amount of carbohydrates you are eating at each meal and snack. It is used intensely by many people with type 1 diabetes to set the appropriate insulin doses for the food they eat.

Here's how it works: Carbohydrate in foods is measured in grams (g). One carb serving is the amount of a food that contains 15 grams of carbohydrate. You can use a kitchen scale to weigh your food, which some people find extremely helpful, especially in the beginning while they're getting familiar with serving sizes. But you can also learn to eyeball it pretty accurately. The rule of thumb is using your fist as a unit measure. Think of your fist as a ball of 15 carbs (as long as your fist isn't unusually large). It's fairly easy to compare a pile of rice or pasta to your fist. If it looks about the size of one fist, it's about 15 grams of carb. Two fists is about 30 grams, and so on.

Pocket Resources

Books and gadgets for understanding carbs are big business these days. In case you're interested in having a little pocket guide that you can easily carry along with you, the ADA offers two: the *Pocket Guide to Diabetic Exchanges* (American Diabetes Association, March 1998) and the *Fast Facts Series Carb Counting Made Easy for People with Diabetes* (American Diabetes Association, 2002). Both are just sixty-four pages of extremely portable and useful information. Getting a feel for the carbohydrate content of your usual foods can be very useful for understanding the impact of your diet on your A1c results.

What Can I Eat?

As we mentioned, most everyone eats healthy foods already. So if you are interested in changing your diet—due to concerns with your A1c, lipids, blood pressure, or weight—you probably don't need to make drastic changes, and you don't need to give up all your favorite foods. What you may need to do is (1) increase the frequency of some of the foods you're already eating, such as vegetables; (2) maybe add or substitute a few new foods, such as using canola oil instead of butter when cooking; and (3) decrease the frequency or portions of some foods that are less beneficial for your present health state, such as brown-bagging your own veggie-rich homemade wrap instead of picking up one stuffed with mystery fillers at the corner deli.

Sugar and Sweeteners

Can you eat sugar if you have diabetes? Nowadays, experts agree that you can, as long as the sugar-containing foods are eaten as part of a balanced meal plan. Sugars are simply carbohydrates, and as long as you keep in mind your total carbohydrate intake, sugars can be part of your diet. High-sugar foods pack in the carbs, and the calories.

Because of this, your portion size of high-sugar foods will need to be small, because these foods are more concentrated in carb. Usually, it's more satisfying to eat a larger portion of a low-sugar breakfast cereal than a tiny portion of a sugary cereal, for example, so factor that in when choosing a sweetened product. Also, many people find high-sugar foods too tempting; it can be hard to stop eating them; it might be best to hold off buying or preparing your favorites, not even having them in the house, except for special treats. A good idea is to look for some agreeable substitutes, rather than trying to give up sweets altogether.

This brings us to sweeteners. What kinds of sweeteners are safe for people with diabetes? There are two kinds: those that contribute calories (called *nutritive* or *caloric* sweeteners) and those that do not (called *nonnutritive* or *noncaloric* sweeteners).

The caloric sweeteners are carbs and do affect your BG levels. Aside from table sugar and sucrose sugars, this category also includes: fructose (fruit sugar), honey, molasses (corn, cane, or date derived), syrups (including agave nectar syrup and brown rice syrup), barley malt, and sugar alcohols. As noted, people with diabetes can consume these—in small amounts and in the context of a balanced diet.

Five non-caloric (and non-carb) sweeteners are now approved by the FDA, meaning they've tested as safe for consumption by the general population:

- **Acesulfame-K** (common brand names: SweetOne, Sunette, Sweet & Safe, Ace-K)
- **Aspartame** (common brand names: NutraSweet, Equal, others)
- **Neotame** (common brand names: not yet available)
- **Saccharin** (common brand names: Sweet 'N Low, Sugar Twin, Necta Sweet, Hermesatas, others)
- **Sucralose** (common brand name: Splenda; watch out for baking varieties that are blended with table sugar, as noted below)

There is no conclusive evidence that any one of these is more or less healthful than another, so it's really up to you to decide on taste. Some are more concentrated than others, and may taste too sweet to your palette.

Note that you cannot totally substitute these noncaloric sweeteners for sugar in baking, because sugar provides a certain bulk that makes the baking process work, and helps to brown the final result. Usually you can replace some of the sugar in a recipe with an artificial sweetener, to at least reduce the overall carbs and calories; the manufacturers of Splenda have introduced part-sugar products specifically for baking.

Fast Food

Fast food restaurants are not only a quick-meal option, they are also everywhere and cheap, and feature menus that beckon you enticingly to the dark side of food. They are perhaps better called "fat food" restaurants because the fare they offer is so high in fat content.

And they take advantage of our love of bargains by offering extra-large (supersize) portions of food at incredibly low prices (often making up the price difference by overcharging for sugary soft drinks, also sold in enormous cups). These massive portions push the total fat, carb, and calorie amounts off the charts of your recommended daily intake. We'd like to say "don't go there," but everyone does at least once in a while. So what can you do to watch your diet? Read on for tips on limiting portion sizes and making sensible substitutions.

Eye on Portion Size

Portion sizes served in restaurants, and at home, have increased steadily over the years. Everything from burgers to muffins to salads are now served in gigantic quantities, often two to three times of what we expected a decade or so ago. Not surprisingly, this increase in portion sizes mirrors the increase of obesity in the United States, especially among young people. Studies show that even people who are not in the habit of finishing all of the food in front of them will still eat more if presented with more. Our perception seems to alter to match the portion size.

This was illustrated in studies directed by food expert and author Dr. Barbara Rolls, in which participants were invited for a series of lunches offering different sizes of sandwiches and chip bags (6- or 12-inch sandwiches, and 1- or 6-ounce bags of chips). They were instructed to eat as much as they wanted, and rate themselves afterward in regard to how hungry or full they felt. Interestingly, when presented with larger portions, the people consumed significantly more calories, but rated themselves afterward almost identically in terms of hunger and fullness, as had those who had eaten smaller portions. On top of that, the folks who ate the larger portions still ate the same number of calories at the next meal. These studies point out the dangers of "supersizing" by showing how easily we can consume extra, unwanted calories—without a natural cap to our sense of hunger kicking in.

Eating out can be tricky this way, because of this tendency to eat more from a plate loaded with giant portions of food. All-you-can-eat buffets are deadly, too, encouraging you to load up your plate with extra servings you don't really need, because the food seems like such a bargain. At home, you have more control, and you might consider limiting your portion sizes by using one of several "plate" methods. For example, the **50-50 Plate Rule** says you should fill half of your plate with high-fiber foods like fruit, fibrous vegetables, and grains, and the other half should be split between protein and other vegetables. Wherever you are, you can make the choice to **start with small portions**. Place small portions on your plate (using a smaller plate helps it to look full), eat them, and then take a little breather before deciding whether you are really hungry enough to go back for a refill.

We also tend to eat food more by visual volume than by actual measurement by weight or calorie content. That is, we tend to eyeball the portion size we're used to eating, and the steady trend toward overly generous servings has made us believe they represent the correct quantities to eat, without really knowing how much comprises a healthy serving for the various nutritional factors we need.

An additonal problem with foods high in fats, such as fast foods, is that they can pack a lot of calories into even a small amount of food. But you can use the flip side of this to your advantage: Try starting your meal with foods that are lower in calorie density, like salads or brothy soups. Studies show that this will decrease your hunger right away, therefore decreasing your overall calorie consumption at that meal. It's important that you do not restrict yourself to the point where you feel frustrated or continuously hungry, as this means you will be less successful in the long run. So for example, if you do give in to the urge of stopping by that burger place, try ordering a salad and a bottle of water first. Only when both have been consumed, decide whether you really need that multipatty burger and a supersize portion of fries, or if smaller portions will give you your flavor fix for both, with perhaps a small diet soda. This way, you fill up on something healthy, and still get to taste the fattier, sweeter foods you crave.

LET YOURSELF EAT

TYING YOURSELF TO a restrictive diet regimen can be hard to manage and even unhealthy:

1. It's not sustainable over time. We all know how hard it is to keep denying ourselves the foods we like. Often dieting ends in binging, or creates a roller-coaster cycle of eating.
2. It's not beneficial for your health. Any method of eating that goes to extremes (for example, the Grapefruit Diet, the Cabbage Soup Diet, the Papaya Diet) deprives your body of other essential substances that it also needs.

Portions can be particularly hard to control at restaurants. Here are some strategies you can use to prevent overeating with the increasing large portions delivered to your table or in takeout deliveries:

- Share a meal.
- Divide your food before you start to eat, and ask to have the rest of it packed to take home in a "doggie bag" to enjoy as a second meal later.
- Create a meal of several appetizers rather than one giant entrée.
- Request that fish or chicken be grilled "dry," without sauces or breading; or your vegetables steamed rather than served in a sauce or butter. More and more chefs are accustomed to complying with this request, so don't be embarrassed to state your preferred cooking method.
- Ask for your sauce or dressing on the side, so that you have more control over how much of it you eat.
- Ask whether the chef can create a fresh fruit dessert for you that contains no sauces or creams.
- At a set-menu dinner, realize that you do not have to eat every course, just because it has been placed in front of you.

- Avoid buffets at restaurants and company dinners, as these tend to encourage us to pile too much food on our plates.

With regard to buffets, we also have some interesting research. Studies by Dr. Rolls and her associates have shown that if people are allowed to eat freely from two different buffets—one with a limited variety of foods, and one with a large variety of foods—they will eat more from the buffet with the larger variety. Sometimes it is helpful to have a snack before arriving at the restaurant, so your choices are not guided by an urgent sense of hunger. (Note that not eating during the day so that you can enjoy your evening meal or a buffet at a special function increases your chance of overindulgence.)

You need to be realistic; nobody is perfect, and beating yourself up with guilt if you overindulge is not likely to help you to choose more sensibly next time. If it's truly a special occasion, it might be reasonable to indulge a *little*—just as long as your "special occasions" do not happen weekly, and you eat healthfully around the iffier foods that you desire, such choosing a salad entrée when you know you'll want a small serving of your favorite pie for dessert.

When you have diabetes, *striking a balance* is everything. Your body needs a variety of foods in moderate amounts. And eating should be enjoyable.

Calculating portion sizes

To learn how to estimate healthy portion sizes, you may need to begin by actually weighing and measuring your food. This will train your eye to gauge portions so you can achieve better glucose control along with weight control:

- Use measuring cups and spoons or a kitchen scale. For accuracy, always weigh cooked food *after* it's cooked (because cooking can alter the food's weight by adding or removing moisture).
- Use a food scale that measures in ounces for weighing foods like meat, poultry, fish, and cheese.

- Use a dry measuring cup for portioning out dry foods like cereal, pasta, and rice.
- Use a liquid measuring cup (shaped like a little pitcher, with a lip for pouring) for liquids like milk and juice.
- Use measuring spoons (not regular eating spoons) for foods taken in smaller amounts, like peanut butter, mayonnaise, oils, and salad dressing.

With practice, you'll learn to eyeball your portions, and won't need to bother measuring familiar foods anymore. The "Visual Portion Sizes" chart may be helpful for staying on-track even away from home and your measuring equipment.

VISUAL PORTION SIZES

BASED ROUGHLY ON an average-size woman's hand:
- Your fist is about the size of 1 cup
- Your palm is about the size of 3 ounces of cooked meat
- Your thumb is about 1 ounce of cheese, or 1 tablespoon of salad dressing or peanut butter
- Your thumb tip is about 1 teaspoon (1 teaspoon = 1 serving of fat, such as butter, margarine, mayonnaise, or oil)
- Your handful is about 1 to 2 ounces of a snack food (a closed handful, not a healping, open handful)

Of picture the following:
- 1 ounce of meat looks like a matchbox
- 1 ounce of cheese is about the size of a Ping-Pong ball
- 1 tablespoon of peanut butter is about the size of a walnut
- 1 cup of fruit is about the size of a baseball
- 1 medium-size apple or orange is about the size of a tennis ball
- 1 portion of clustered grapes (a 1/2-cup serving) is about the size of a light bulb
- A medium-size potato is about the size of a computer mouse

If you eat away from home a lot, it's easy to get lazy and lose sight of portion sizes. So when you are at home, it's a good idea to make the effort to go back periodically to weighing and measuring your food, to keep your portion estimation skills strong.

What's a Balanced Meal?

So now you've got the idea of limiting portion size. But how do you determine how many portions of what you're supposed to eat each day? The FDA's Food Pyramid gives general recommendations:

- 6 or more servings of grains, beans and starchy vegetables
- 2 to 3 servings of milk products
- 2 to 3 servings of meat and other protein
- 3 to 5 servings of nonstarchy vegetables
- 2 to 4 servings of fruit
- Limited quantities of fats, sweets, and alcohol

You may also be wondering what a balanced meal looks like. Essentially this means a meal that contains all or at least several of the key food components listed above—carb, protein, fiber, and possibly a little fat. The trouble is that so many of our typical meals contain far too much fat, and almost all carb: sweetened cereal plus toast and juice; lo mein or fried rice with fried dumplings; spaghetti with garlic bread. These are all examples of meals that are nearly *all carb*.

Achieving balance means learning to mix up your food choices a little. It helps to keep thinking about places where you can swap a healthy protein or fiber choice for those high-carb items. For example, instead of breakfast cereal with toast and juice, try scrambled eggs with a little fruit and yogurt on the side. For lunch, order a steamed vegetable dish with brown rice on the side. Or for dinner, instead of pasta with garlic bread, try a lean meat accompanied by a salad and a slice of bread or two (not more).

Food Choices for Your Personal Health Needs

Eating to Lower Your A1c

Overall portion size, and in particular the quantity of carbohydrates you eat, are key here. Fats and proteins do affect your BG, but carbohydrates have the main effect. A common mistake is to think that this means you can't or shouldn't eat carbohydrates, since they raise your BG. But remember: your BG is high not because of carbohydrates, but because you have diabetes.

Carbohydrates are your body's essential fuel, and in most diets should make up the bulk of your food. General recommendations (from the American Diabetes Association and other government health organizations) say that for people with diabetes, carbs should still make up 40 to 60 percent of the daily calories you consume. An easy way to calculate this is to divide the number of calories in your daily diet by 8, which produces the number of grams of carbohydrate you should eat each day. For example, if you are consuming about 2,000 calories each day, divide that by 8 and you get the number of grams of carbohydrate you should be eating, which is 250 grams. This would account for 50 percent (exactly half) of your daily calories.

Ten percent higher or lower would give you the carbohydrate grams for 40 and 60 percent, which would be 225 grams and 275 grams, respectively. This would give you an average of 75 grams of carb per meal (225 divided by 3 meals per day) or more.

To understand more about carbohydrates and type 2 diabetes, it helps to remember (or learn if you haven't already) the physiology underlying your diabetes. Type 2 diabetes results from two changes in your body: an inefficient insulin secretion response to glucose, and a resistance to the effects of the insulin that is present. Put simply, this means that too many carbohydrates can overwhelm your sluggish insulin response system. This also explains why it's useful for you to spread your carbohydrates (your main fuel) throughout the day, including your all-important first meal of the day, breakfast. Eating breakfast jump-starts your energy and your metabolism (your body's food-processing system) for the day.

If you are taking insulin, then you'll need to follow your carbo-hydrate intake even more closely, using one of two general approaches: either by (1) eating a consistent amount of carbohy-drates at each meal, or (2) counting your carbs and then using an insulin-to-carbohydrate ratio to set insulin doses for each meal. By "consistent carbohydrates," we mean that every day at breakfast, you have about the same amount of carbs as you eat at every other breakfast. Lunches may have a different amount of carb from breakfast, but will need to stay the same amount from one lunch to the next. The same goes for dinner each day. The types and forms of carbs may vary, but the total amount of eaten at each meal-time needs to be consistent. Using this approach, if you sometimes have a sandwich and a fruit for lunch (a healthy choice) and some-times have a chicken Caesar salad (also a healthy choice, especially with the dressing on the side), you will be creating an insulin-carbohydrate misbalance—since the one lunch has considerably more carbs than the other. The sandwich and fruit are mostly carbs, while the chicken Caesar has none except for the croutons.

If you are taking insulin and want some flexibility in the amount of carbs you eat from one lunch to another, you will need to use carb counting (see page 131), and then calculate how much insulin you need at each meal based on your insulin-to-carb ratio. This ratio varies from person to person, so you will need your doctor's or diabetes educator's help to determine your personal ratio. But, for example, if your ratio was 1 to 15, you would take 1 unit of insulin for every 15 grams of carbohydrate that you eat.

By controlling your carbohydrate intake, you will have taken your first step toward controlling your A1c. Once you have set a con-sistent and reasonable amount of carbs in your diet, any further improvements in your A1c will need to come from increased phys-ical activity, or a change in medication, or both.

Eating to Lower Your Lipid Levels

The types of fat you eat have a major effect on your lipid levels. Although all fats pack the same number of calories, and have the same effect on your weight, they vary greatly in their effect on your cholesterol and cardiovascular risk. If your LDL is high and/or your HDL is low, eating less saturated and trans fats, and more polyunsaturated and monounsaturated fats, will move your numbers into a better range.

Fat-Rich Foods to Avoid
- Beef and pork (select only lean cuts when you do eat them)
- Poultry skin
- Palm oil and coconut oil—look for these ingredients on food labels
- Whole milk and cheeses, and cream-style sauces

Fat-Rich Foods to Choose
- Canola, olive, safflower and sunflower, corn, and peanut oils
- Nuts such as almonds and walnuts
- Fish, especially salmon, trout, and swordfish, which are high in omega-3 fats

A QUICK GUIDE TO FATS

TYPE OF FAT	EFFECT	RECOMMENDATION	SOURCES
Saturated fat	Raises cholesterol	Up to 7% of calories	Fatty meat, whole milk, poultry skin
Trans fat	Raises cholesterol	Avoid	Commercial baked goods, snacks, fast and convenience foods, solid shortening, palm and coconut oil
Monounaturated fat	Lowers cholesterol	Up to 20% of calories	Olive, soy, and canola oil
Polyunsaturated fat	Lowers cholesterol	Up to 10% of calories	Other oils (except for palm and coconut oil), salad dressings
Omega-3 fat	Heart-healthy	Eat more	Fish, fish oil supplements, omega-3-enriched eggs

In addition to changing the types of fats you eat, eating foods that contain soluble, or *viscous*, fiber (oats and barley, eggplant and okra) or adding soluble fiber in the form of *psyllium* (Metamucil, Fiberall, Effersyllium, and others) will also help lower your LDL cholesterol. Substances called *plant-sterols*, which are present in some enriched margarines, also have a cholesterol-lowering effect. Some studies have shown that diets including these components, along with healthy nuts such as walnuts and almonds, are as effective as low doses of statin drugs in lowering your LDL. Remember, statin medications are not meant to replace the effects of your diet changes, but rather to *reinforce* to the LDL-lowering effects of the foods you choose.

KNOW YOUR FAT SOURCES

THIS TABLE SHOWS the types of fat contained in 1 table-spoon of each source, listed in grams. One tablespoon of any fat has about 120 calories, so use just a little, please.

Also note that your better choices are at the top of the table; those further down the list contain increasing amounts of "bad fat."

SOURCE	SATURATED	MONOUNSATURATED	POLYUNSATURATED	OTHER
Safflower oil	0.8	10.2	2.0	0.6
Canola oil	1.0	8.2	4.1	0.7
Flaxseed oil	1.3	2.5	10.2	0.0
Sunflower oil	1.4	2.7	8.9	0.6
Corn oil	1.7	3.3	8.0	0.6
Olive oil	1.8	10.0	1.2	0.5
Sesame oil	1.9	5.4	5.6	0.7
Soybean oil	2.0	3.2	7.8	0.6
Peanut oil	2.3	6.2	4.3	0.7
Cottonseed oil	3.5	2.4	7.0	0.7
Chicken fat	3.8	5.7	2.6	0.7
Lard (pork fat)	5.0	5.8	1.4	0.6
Beef fat	6.4	5.4	0.5	0.5
Palm oil	6.7	5.0	1.2	0.7
Butter	7.2	3.3	0.5	0.5
Cocoa butter	8.1	4.5	0.4	0.6
Palm kernel oil	11.1	1.6	0.2	0.7
Coconut oil	11.8	0.8	0.2	0.8

Eating to Lower Your Blood Pressure

Several things in your diet can impact your blood pressure. One "dash" of knowledge here comes from the Dietary Approaches to Stop Hypertension (DASH) clinical studies. These multicenter national studies looked at the effects of eating increased amounts of fruits and vegetables on lowering blood pressure. The DASH diets included 2 to 2.5 cups of fruit and 2 to 2.5 cups of vegetables every day, along with 4 to 5 servings per week of nuts, seeds, and dried beans. These fruits and vegetables help lower blood pressure, and also contain phytonutrients that have many other health benefits as well. You can learn more about the DASH diet at the National Institute of Health Web site, www.nhlbi.nih.gov/health/public/heart/hbp/dash/.

Sodium

When it comes to salt intake, some individuals with high blood pressure are much more sensitive to its effects than others. Salt intake includes table salt that you add yourself, plus the sodium present in prepared foods. It is this second source that often causes the problem. Processed foods, including frozen foods like frozen dinners, can contain surprisingly high amounts of sodium, even though they don't necessarily taste salty. Remember that sodium may also be used as a preservative, as a leavening agent in the form of baking soda (sodium bicarbonate) or baking powder (sodium bicarbonate plus either tartaric acid or sodium aluminum sulfate), as an additive in cured foods such as smoked fish and hot dogs (sodium nitrate and nitrite), or as a dough conditioner (sodium stearyl lactylate or sodium stearyl fumarate); all these variations must be listed in a product's ingredient list and contribute to its overall sodium score. The FDA's recommended daily amount is less than 2,300 mg of sodium (or 2.3 grams, about 1 teaspoon of table salt). If your blood pressure is sensitive to sodium, you will benefit from lowering your sodium intake to 1,500 mg/day. If you miss adding salt to your foods, you can achieve this flavor by using spices and non-sodium-chloride salt substitutes.

TASTE SENSATIONS

EACH ONE OF us has five different taste receptors in our mouths, mostly on our tongue:

- salty
- sour
- sweet
- bitter
- umami, a savory protein taste exemplified by glutamate, including monosodium glutamate (MSG)

Most of our different taste sensations are a combination of these five receptors, plus texture. The "sweet" receptor, as you might guess, is very potent, and mammals can't seem to get enough of it. Consider what a bear goes through to get to honey in the wild!

Potassium chloride, for one, is marketed as an alternative salt (and has no negative effects on your blood pressure). More and more reduced-salt products are being offered, such as low-sodium soy sauce and ketchup. It's also true that you can train yourself to appreciate a slightly salty taste without needing large amounts of it; your number of salt receptors can actually increase slightly as you eat less salt, so that you taste small quantities more vividly.

Eating to Reduce Your Weight

We left this to last, since weight loss is clearly a difficult area. If there were a simple, easy way to lose weight, everyone would be doing it. If you think that just eating less is simple, you haven't looked at all the research clearly telling us that this is far from the truth. Losing weight is not simple to accomplish, and even harder to maintain.

Patients have in fact lost weight in hundreds of different diet studies, but one common result is that the weight loss isn't maintained, as staying on any of these diets for longer than a few months is difficult at best. Diet studies that don't include an exercise component show even less success in maintaining weight loss. The studies also show that the amount of weight lost is almost always due to eating less calories overall—even with diets such as the Atkin's low-carb diet, that do not specifically address or count calories. What this means is that it's not the carb-reduction that helps you lose weight, but rather the direct effect of eating carefully and therefore eating less while dieting. Despite claims about "fat-burning," or changing your metabolism, the general laws of thermodynamics hold, and you can't lose weight without eating fewer calories. This may sound gloomy, but we know that many people are successful in losing weight, and keeping it off. Researchers recently started the National Weight Control Registry for monitoring just such people. They have found several common factors in those who have lost significant amounts of weight and kept it off.

Most significantly, on average, these people continue to exercise daily for more than an hour each day, averaging over 3,000 calories a week of energy burned. (Most gym equipment gives you an approximation of the calories burned during your exercise; walking at a fast pace on flat ground is about 360 calories per hour). Although their individual diets vary, all the registrants monitor their weight and food consumption regularly, and their diets tend to be low in fat. Another common factor is a piece of advice your mother probably gave you: they tend to eat breakfast regularly.

What about fad diets, then, and the advertisements for weight-loss products you see on TV? As far as supplements and "fat-burners" go, they have no proven benefit for weight loss. Remember that dietary supplements are not regulated by the FDA, so the vendors can make any claims they like without real evidence to back them up. Although the Federal Trade Commission (FTC) occasionally intervenes in the case of outrageous claims, this is rare. The reason many of these diets are initially successful is because of restrictions to certain foods, or the use of a diuretic (which causes you to lose excess water weight). Fewer choices usually means people eat fewer calories, but it also means that the diet will be difficult to maintain, and perhaps worse: an unbalanced diet could lead to a reduced intake of necessary nutrients, especially those in fruits and vegetables. Water loss, meanwhile, washes nutrients out of your body before they can be used.

The secret to healthy and successful weight loss is eating a variety of food types, while burning more calories than you are taking in.

Healthy Eating for Everyone

WHAT WE'VE DESCRIBED here in this chapter is healthy eating for anyone, with or without diabetes. And when it comes to diet and weight issues, there are three important things that everyone should keep in mind:

1. **There's a big difference between what is a healthy weight for you, and some idealized vision you or others have of being thin.** Our culture tends to idolize people with a slim frame, and movies and advertising sometimes glamorize this to the point of making the rest of us feel ugly and unwanted. But this is just fashion, not health.

2. **If you regularly exercise and eat healthful foods in reasonable amounts, and your weight remains steady, then chances are you don't need to make any food changes, even if your body is a little more "round" than most bodies you see on TV.** Your challenge is not to master a regimen that promises miraculous weight loss, but rather to accept your body's basic shape for what it is, and use exercise not to remove but to tone what is there.

3. **The intensity with which you do decide to make food changes should be guided by your Diabetes Health Account.** If you have some health debts, you'll want to use diet changes as a tool for addressing those, as outlined in this chapter.

As we've mentioned often in this book, your dietary changes don't have to be drastic. You may only need to start with a single immediate change, for example adding more fruits and vegetables to your diet. If your Diabetes Health Account is in good shape, then you can relax and think about slower, longer-term changes that will gradually make your diet as healthful as possible.

9 Diabetes Drugs:
What Are They and What Do They Do?

OUR GOAL IN this chapter is to tell you everything you need to know about the medications that affect your diabetes, and then some. Obviously, you'll want to read closely the sections most pertinent for you, and perhaps skim others out of interest. The very curious will want to read it all. But before plunging into the specifics of thiazolidinediones (a word that only endocrinologists can pronounce without a struggle), let's take a step back and look at the bigger picture.

Needing Drugs Doesn't Mean Your Diabetes Is "Worse"

FOR MANY PATIENTS WITH type 2 diabetes, two of their primary goals are: (1) avoiding insulin, and (2) taking as few pills as possible. A typical thought process goes like this: "I know I can do this myself if I just work harder," "I don't want to use the pills as a crutch," "I know what to do; I just need to eat better and start exercising." Sound familiar? These are common statements and beliefs, but they show a basic misunderstanding of the impact of diabetes, and are likely to lead to greater frustration and poorer outcomes in the long-term.

We know that everyone who has diabetes is different, that your diabetes is different from that of most other people, and that you bring your own strengths and weaknesses into the struggle with the disease. Despite these differences, there are two common facts that apply to everyone. First, one of your goals, even if you have not specifically stated it, is to lead a long and healthy life with diabetes. The second fact is that your diabetes itself changes over time; its genes induce changes inside your body that progress, causing a slow decrease in the capacity of your pancreas to secrete insulin, and, in some cases, create a further increase in insulin resistance. This rate of progression varies between individuals, and you can slow the progress, but you can't prevent it. This progression of the disease inside your body *does not* mean that you are doomed to complications, or that your attempts to control your diabetes have failed. Rather, it means that because of the very nature of the disease itself, you may need to change your diabetes regimen over time, to adjust to the inevitable changes in insulin secretion and insulin resistance.

In short, you need to revisit the lessons of chapter 2. Your diabetes is not "worse" if you have to take pills, or if you eventually take insulin. Your diabetes *is* "worse," however, if despite all your best efforts to watch your diet and exercise, your A1c is higher. You need to keep your eye on your A1c result, not on the treatment needed to achieve it. Someone with an A1c of 8.2 who is controlling his BG with exercise and diet only has a higher risk of complications than someone who is taking two diabetes pills, but who has an A1c of 7.0. In fact, this second patient will have 30 percent lower chance of diabetes-related complications, because of the pills.

So, keeping in mind that your A1c is the primary indicator of your glucose control, what do you do when your A1c is above target, even though you're doing as well as you possibly can with lifestyle interventions? The answer lies in a phased approach to glucose control. In its purest form, this means adding a diabetes pill to your present regimen of activity and food, then increasing the dose, then adding a second type of diabetes pill, then increasing that dose, and so on. The final stage after taking two different types of diabetes pills is either adding a third type, or switching to insulin.

As mentioned, many patients view this progression of treatment as a failure on their part; they feel guilty about not having made sufficient lifestyle changes, or "know" that if they just tried harder, they wouldn't need the assistance of diabetes pills. Though understandable, these feelings are medical nonsense. Remember, diabetes is a genetic disease, and its tendency to progress over time comes with the package. Period. Your job is to adjust your diabetes regimen to keep ahead of this process, working to maintain your A1c goal by whatever combination of treatments is most practical at any given point in time. By focusing on your A1c results rather than your treatment, you will be able to outlive your diabetes and hopefully shake the guilt syndrome.

The Main Classes of Medications

FOUR MAIN CLASSES of medications have been used for many years to lower BGs, and two more classes just came out in 2004., There are three main categories of pills specifically for type 2 diabetes. Each category works through a separate mechanism, so that their effects are additive. These categories work equally well in lowering your A1c.

Sulfonylureas and Their Cousins

Sulfonylureas were the first oral medications found to have an effect on lowering BG. They were discovered in the 1940s, as researchers followed up on findings that sulfonamides, early antibiotics used in World War II, produced low BGs in some patients. Scientists soon produced modifications of sulfonamides that had consistent effects on lowering BG, and sulfonylureas were born. The early sulfonylureas (*tolbutamide, chlorpropamide, acetohexamide,* and *tolazamide*) were replaced in the 1970s by newer agents, which could be taken in smaller doses, with fewer side effects. Today, there are three commonly used medications in this class: *glipizide*, *glipuride*, and *glimeperide*.

Method of action

The primary action of these medications is to stimulate the insulin-producing cells in your pancreas to secrete more insulin, resulting in lower BGs. They also have other actions, not well understood, that seem to increase the effectiveness of circulating insulin. Their major effect, though, is to increase the amount of insulin released by your pancreas.

Sulfonylureas increase your insulin levels throughout the day, even when you haven't eaten, and because of this, can sometimes cause low BGs (hypoglycemia). A derivative class of medication, called *meglitanides*, was developed to boost insulin secretion following each meal. This approach is closer to the way the human body normally secretes insulin, but the medications in this class do not have as strong an effect on lowering your A1c, typically bringing it down by less than 1 percent when used alone.

Usage information

GENERIC NAME	TRADE NAME	DOSE RANGE (MG)	DOSES PER DAY
Glipizide	Glucotrol	1.25–20	one or two doses
Glyburide	Micronase, Diabeta	1.25–20	one or two doses
Glimeperide	Amaryl	1–8	one dose
Repaglinide	Prandin	0.5–4	
Nateglinide	Starlix	60–120	

Side effects

The most common side effect is a low risk of hypoglycemia (low BG).

Metformin: In a Class by Itself

Metformin belongs to the biguanides class of drugs, and is the only one in this class available in the United States. In the '70s, another biguanide used in the United States, *phenformin*, was withdrawn from the market because of a side effect called lactic acidosis (a dangerous blood disorder). Because of its similarities to phenformin, metformin wasn't initially marketed in the United States. By 1990, the FDA was finally convinced of the safety and efficacy of this drug, and it has now become the most commonly used oral diabetes medication. Because studies have shown that metformin can reduce weight gain, it is often the first choice of medication for patients with type 2 diabetes, especially if they are overweight.

Method of action

Metformin exerts its major action on the liver. It counteracts the problem of insulin resistance by decreasing release of glucose from the liver. The liver is the body's main metabolic factory, and produces glucose in two ways; by breaking down starches, and by making new glucose molecules directly. Metformin intervenes in both of these pathways.

Usage information

GENERIC NAME	TRADE NAME	DOSE RANGE (MG)	DOSES PER DAY
Metformin	Glucophage, Glucophage XR, Riomet, Fortamet, Glumetza	500 mg to 2,550 mg	Varies (see below)

Metformin is usually taken with meals, as it is less likely to cause abdominal discomfort when taken with food. Occasionally the pill is not fully broken down and absorbed after swallowing. If this occurs, a liquid version is also available.

The lowest starting dose is 500 mg once a day, and the maximum dose is 2,550 mg, taken as 850 mg three times per day. There is also a long-lasting version that can be taken once a day.

Side effects

Metformin's most common side effect is abdominal discomfort: mild nausea, diarrhea, and gas. These symptoms are not common, and if they occur when first starting metformin, they sometimes decrease over a week's time. If the symptoms persist, you should discuss alternatives with your doctor.

A more serious side effect, lactic acidosis, can occur in patients with congestive heart failure or decreased kidney function (a blood creatinine test of 1.4 or higher). Your health-care provider can provide this information for you.

Thiazolidinediones: The Newest and the Best?

Thiazolidinediones (TZDs) are the newest class of glucose-lowering medications, and work on through completely different pathway than the other medications. They reduce insulin resistance in fat cells and muscles, and also have additional, possibly beneficial effects on fat cells and some other hormones. These medications have also been used to treat *polycystic ovary disease* (PCOS), and *lipodystrophy*, which are other diseases sometimes associated with insulin resistance.

The first TZD that came to market, *troglitazone* (Rezulin) was subsequently withdrawn when the newer TZDs became available. The original version caused severe liver damage in a very small number of patients. Because of this, later forms, *pioglitazone* and *rosiglitazone*, were carefully monitored for liver toxicity, but neither has been found to have similar negative effects.

Method of action

The TZDs exert their major action on reducing insulin resistance through a pathway involving *peroxisome proliferators-activated receptors* (PPAR). These receptors reside in the cell nucleus, and bind fatty acids and other molecules. TZDs compete for this binding, and this results in a number of effects, including increased glucose uptake by your cells. There are also interesting effects on fat cell development and on the release of hormones produced by fat cells, which are still being studied by researchers.

Usage information

GENERIC NAME	TRADE NAME	DOSE RANGE (MG)	DOSES PER DAY
Pioglitazone	Actos	15 to 45	Once a day
Rosiglitazone	Avandia	4 to 8	Once a day

Side effects

Fluid retention is one side effect of this class of drug, which can result in some weight gain. Because of this, these medications should be used very carefully or not at all if you have congestive heart failure, or a risk for congestive heart failure. Caution should be used if you already have problems with edema, or swelling of your legs.

Occasionally these medications can affect the liver, causing an increase in liver function tests, such as the ALT. Because of this, you should have your ALT checked before starting these medications, and periodically (once or twice a year) afterward. If your ALT rises to more than 2½ times the upper limit of normal, your healthcare provider should suggest switching to another medication or reducing your dose.

Alpha-Glucosidase Inhibitors

These medications, which include *acarbose* and *miglitol*, are used more commonly in Canada and Europe than the United States. They have a unique mode of action, in that they are not absorbed into your blood, but work directly in your gut, or intestines.

Method of action

Alpha-glucosidase is an enzyme that breaks down more complex sugar molecules into simpler glucose molecules (*monosaccharides*), which are then absorbed from your gut into your blood. Inhibiting this enzyme delays the breakdown and absorption of carbohydrates, decreasing the rise in glucose following a meal, and lowering your overall BGs. What actually happens is that the carbohydrates travel further down your gut before they are completely digested and absorbed. In most people, the bacteria present deeper in the gut are different than those present at the entryway to the intestines. When these deeper bacteria encounter the carbohydrates, they are transformed into fuel.

Usage information

GENERIC NAME	TRADE NAME	DOSE RANGE (MG)	DOSES PER DAY
Acarbose	Precose	25–100	With the start of each meal
Miglitol	Glyset	25–100	With the start of each meal

Since their effect is on delaying absorption of the carbohydrates you eat, these medicines need to be taken just as you begin eating, together with your first bite of food.

If you have a low BG episode while taking one of these medications, you need to treat it with some *pure* form of glucose, such as glucose tablets or gel. Other treatments won't work, since common sugars such as sucrose and lactose are *disaccharides*, whose break-down and absorption are prevented by alpha-glucosidase inhibitors.

Side effects

The major side effect is abdominal discomfort and production of increased amounts of gas, which can result in increased flatu-lence. Your intestines are normally full of bacteria that help aid in breaking down your food. Your body usually breaks down and absorbs most carbohydrates before reaching the bacteria further down in your gut, which species often produce gas when exposed to carbohydrates. Using alpha-glucosidase blockers delays the digestion and absorption of carbohydrates, so these deeper bacte-ria are exposed to more carbohydrates, and produce more gas.

This is a temporary effect. As time goes by, the bacteria in your body adapts to the new situation: the bacteria present at the entry-way to your gut, which don't produce the gas, move further down your intestines, following the supply of carbohydrates. This bac-terial emigration can then cause a decrease in gas and side effects.

Insulins: Always a Good Choice

Insulin is a simple medicine, complicated by common misper-ceptions. It is one of only a few medications that are completely natural. That is, we can give insulin as a "medication" that is exactly the same as the insulin humans already have present in their bodies, circulating in their blood. This means you don't need to worry about any side effects, or unusual reactions to insulin as a medication. The only concerns related to insulin are in the results: if too little insulin is given, your BGs and your A1c will be too high; if too much insulin is given, your BG may go too low, caus-ing you to have an unpleasant hypoglycemic episode. But make no mistake: today's human insulins offer one of the best treatments available for controlling BG.

In the past, the insulin used for treating diabetes came from pigs and cows, and was purified in pharmaceutical plants. Pure human insulin first became available in 1982. This was made possible by the discovery and sequencing of the human insulin gene. The genetic sequence was duplicated, and this human gene placed into either special bacteria or yeast, which produce large amounts of human insulin. This can easily be collected and purified.

The difficulty, of course, is in administering insulin in the same way that your body does naturally. People without diabetes constantly secrete low levels of insulin to cover their basic metabolic needs. Even when you are not eating, your body needs a basic background, or *basal* amount of insulin. This allows glucose—the common fuel for your body's cells—to leave your blood and enter the cells. In addition, your pancreas also secretes short bursts of insulin during meals, to help store away the food-induced increases in glucose. This type of insulin secretion, in response to a meal, is called a *bolus* of insulin.

The challenge is, therefore, administer insulin via a needle, pump, or other device, in a way that most closely replicates the body's basal and bolus needs.

Method of action

Insulin is a type of protein called a *hormone*, which means it is secreted by an organ in the body directly into the blood stream, and then has an effect on distant cells. In a healthy human body, the insulin is secreted by a group of cells called *islets*, which are scattered throughout your pancreas. Although housed in the pancreas, the islets are functionally separate—and even comprise a physically separate organ in a few species, like in certain types of fish. The rest of the pancreas produces enzymes that are secreted through into the small intestine, where they aid in the digestion of the carbohydrates, fats, and proteins that you eat.

The distant cells affected by insulin are in the liver, muscle, and fatty tissue. These cells contain insulin receptors on their surface; when your circulating insulin passes by one of these receptors, it becomes attached, in a tight fit, similar to a key fitting into a lock. The insulin receptor stretches from the outside to the inside of the cell, triggering the "lock" inside of the cell to turn automatically.

A cascade of events then occurs inside the cell, including the increased transportation of glucose into the cell. This transportation is important for two reasons. The most immediate is that your cells then have glucose available as a fuel, and are able to function normally. The second is that excess glucose is removed from your circulating blood. As you well know by now, this is important over the longer term because high levels of glucose in your blood (identified by high A1c results), are associated with an increased likelihood of diabetes-related complications in the future.

The different insulins used to treat diabetes vary in their time course of action. Some are designed for rapid action at mealtimes, some for long-lasting effect overnight, and others for a middle ground. They can be used individually or in combination. Some of the variation in action is also due to varied rates of absorption from the injection site—your stomach usually absorbs a shot faster than your thigh, for example. Once these insulins are absorbed into your blood, they work quickly and similarly to each other.

Usage information

GENERIC NAME	TRADE NAME	MINUTES UNTIL ONSET	DURATION IN HOURS
Aspart	Novolog	10–45	3–6
Glulisine	Apidra	10–45	3–6
Lispro	Humalog	10–45	3–6
Regular	Humulin, Novolin	30–90	4–8
NPH	Humulin N, Novolin N	120–480	8–24 (some peak)
Detemir	Levemir	60–120	12–24 (no peak)
Glargine	Lantus	60–120	20–24 (no peak)

In contrast to other medications, insulin has no real dosage limits; adjustments are made based on your carbohydrate intake, current BG results, and A1c.

Faster-acting insulin (lispro, aspart, glulisine, and Regular) should be taken before meals, preferably just before eating. Regular insulin may have a better effect if taken 15 to 20 minutes in advance of a meal.

Longer-acting insulins (NPH, glargine, and detemir) are taken once or twice a day, usually in the morning or at bedtime. Because of their slower course of action, they don't need to be taken in any particular relation to food.

Side effects

As mentioned, insulin itself does not in itself cause any unrelated side effects. The main caution lies in proper dosing: too high or too low BG values can result when your insulin regimen is not properly balanced with other factors in your everyday life, such as diet and degree of activity.

Low BG episodes are easily treated, with 15 grams of simple (fast-acting) carbohydrate. They are less likely to occur, and easier to detect and treat, in patients with type 2 diabetes compared to patients with type 1.

Some people, including health-care providers, worry about the possibility of weight gain when taking insulin. The effect of insulin on weight gain was best shown during the United Kingdom Prospective Diabetes Study (UKPDS), in which more than 4,000 patients with type 2 diabetes were followed for over ten years on different treatments. Compared to sulfonylureas, treatment with insulin was associated with an increased weight gain of about 4½ pounds over ten years. Although this difference is significant, the amount is relatively small, and not nearly enough to outweigh the benefits of insulin treatment.

Incretins

This is a brand new class of drugs, the first of which became widely available in 2005. *Incretins* are intestinal hormones long studied for their variety of effects on glucose metabolism that are relevant to diabetes. The best understood of these hormones, *glucagon-like polypeptide 1* (GLP-1), is extremely short-acting, so researchers studying it have needed to give it intravenously. As a diabetes treatment, it is digested too quickly when taken by mouth, and therefore must be given by injection, similar to insulin.

Surprisingly, a similar substance was discovered in the saliva of Gila monsters, and had the advantage of a much longer period of action. You may have heard of the first drug based on this substance, now available in an injection pen: Byetta.

Method of action

Incretins have several distinct actions that are beneficial for patients with type 2 diabetes. They increase insulin secretion, in a manner not completely understood but functionally different from the effects of high glucose—which triggers insulin secretion in a healthy body. Incretins also decrease the secretion of *glucagon*, a hormone produced in the pancreatic islets and elsewhere, that raises BG (to oppose the effects of insulin). In addition, incretins delay gastric emptying, which in layman's terms means your food is digested more slowly. This may account for the sustained weight loss that patients often experience, one of the enticing effects of incretin treatment. Another very promising effect of incretins is that they seem to promote the growth of islet cells, shown in research with animals. Although researchers haven't been able to demonstrate this effect yet in people (as of 2006), the possibility of increasing your body's own supply of insulin is quite exciting.

Usage information

GENERIC NAME	TRADE NAME	DOSE RANGE (MCG)	DOSES PER DAY
Exenatide	Byetta	5 mcg (micrograms) twice a day; can be increased to 10 mcg after the patient adjusts to changes in digestion	Given by injection twice a day, usually morning and evening

We expect other forms of incretin therapy to enter the market by 2007, offering additional benefits. A long-lasting, once-a-week form of exenatide (exenatide LAR) is currently being tested, as well as a once-a-day version called liraglutide. These new forms will last longer in your body by suppressing certain enzymes and hormones.

Your natural incretin, GLP-1, is broken down in your body by an enzyme called dipeptidyl peptidase-IV (DPP-IV). Inhibiting this enzyme would allow your own internal GLP-1 to last longer and have a greater effect. Vidagliptin and Sitagliptin are two other glucose-reducing drugs, called *DPP-IV inhibitors*, currently under study. In addition to prolonging your GLP-1, the DPP-IV inhibitors also inhibit the breakdown of another gut hormone called glucose-dependent insulinotropic peptide (GIP), which may account for some differences between their effects and those of incretins, such as less effect on weight loss. These medicines will likely be making headlines in the future, so keep your eyes peeled, and ask your health-care provider about any news.

Side effects

Nausea is the most common side effect. Low BGs can also occur, especially when used with other hypoglycemia-causing medications.

Amylin Analogs

Amylin is a naturally occurring hormone produced in the islets, the same cells that produce insulin. Though it was discovered over a decade ago, its main functions and metabolic importance are still unknown. Although similar to incretins (such as exenatide) in some of its effects, it is structurally different, and does not belong to the same family. Like many other hormones, amylin has a short duration of action, and researchers studying its action needed to give it intravenously. Longer acting analogs have now become available.

Method of action

Unlike the incretins, amylin analogs do not increase insulin secretion. Their main effect may be in delaying gastric emptying, which delays the rise in glucose following meals. They also decrease the secretion of glucagon, and seem to decrease appetite. Early studies have shown some weight loss in patients taking amylin analogs.

Usage information

GENERIC NAME	TRADE NAME	DOSE RANGE (MCG)	DOSES PER DAY
Pramlintide	Symlin	Starting dose is 60 mcg (micrograms), and is increased every three days until nausea occurs, or a dose of 120 mcg is reached	Given by injection (similar to insulin) before each meal

This drug is injected with an insulin syringe, but cannot be mixed with insulin. Your doctor will usually reduce the dose of your insulin when starting pramlintide to reduce risk of resulting low BGs. When the maximum tolerated dose of Symlin is reached, the insulin can be increased again if necessary.

Side effects

The most common side effect is nausea, which often limits the maximum dose that can be taken. Since it slows gastric emptying, patients taking other medications that affect gastric emptying should not take pramlintide. Patients with an uncommon complication of diabetes that causes this condition, known as *delayed gastric motility* (*gastroparesis*), should also avoid this medication.

10 Understanding Hypo- and Hyperglycemia

Fear of Low Blood Glucose

ONE OF THE scariest aspects of diabetes is the prospect of experiencing low blood glucose. As if to make this situation even a little scarier, physicians call this phenomenon by the intimidating medical term *hypoglycemia*, shortened by diabetes veterans to *hypos*. That really does sound like something to avoid.

But fear alone is pretty useless. So let's learn a little more about low BGs, and what they mean to you. Hypoglycemia is defined as any test result under 70 mg/dL, or under 80 mg/dL with symptoms. In this case, it wasn't a committee that decided on the cutoff point, but your body. This is the point at which your body can no longer function properly, and it makes you feel very uncomfortable: nervous, sweaty, muddle-headed, and/or shaky. When your BG hits levels below 65 to 70, these feelings are caused by the adrenaline your body produces in order to bring the glucose up slightly, and keep it from dropping lower.

Glucose Response in People without Diabetes

To understand why this happens in people with diabetes, it's important to know how things worked before you developed this disease. In people without diabetes, the body has an automatic, self-regulating glucose control system. It works this way: to keep the BG levels in the blood from running too high, the body relies on insulin. Remember that insulin latches on to receptors on the outside of your cells, opening a lock that allows glucose to move from your blood into your muscle, fat, and liver cells. When the BG rises even slightly, the pancreas secretes insulin into the blood, where it acts immediately to move glucose into cells, thus lowering the concentration of glucose in the blood. To keep the glucose levels from falling too low, as it might after a prolonged period without food, the pancreas stops secreting insulin, so that the glucose stays in the blood. The body also automatically counteracts low BG; very low levels of insulin encourage the liver to release glucose from its reserve stores, which keeps the glucose levels from dropping dangerously low.

A healthy body also has two other fast-acting levels of protection from hypoglycemia. When the BG falls below 70 (at which point insulin output is halted), two other hormones are quickly released: *glucagon* and *epinephrine*. Glucagon is a hormone that directly counteracts many of the actions of insulin. It raises BG by increasing glucose release from the liver, from muscle cells, and even from cells in your kidney. Epinephrine also acts through different pathways in these same cells to increase the BG. Glucagon and epinephrine are the immediate second-level of response, and are quite effective.

"SCARY" LOW BLOOD GLUCOSE: FIGHT OR FLIGHT

WHY ARE LOW blood glucose episodes scary?

Epinephrine, also called *adrenaline*, has other effects in addition to raising the BG. It triggers the same adrenaline "fight-or-flight" hormone that your body releases if you are in a frightening situation and need to supercharge your body.

The symptoms include a faster heart rate, increased sensitivity of your nervous system resulting in shaking and sometimes

> goose bumps, and a movement of blood flow from your skin to
> your muscles.
>
> These are important clues that your BG might be low. But
> they also make you feel uncomfortable, and even scared—because
> your body is acting in just the same way it does when you're afraid.

There is also a third, slower response of the body involving two
other hormones that can help raise the BG; *cortisol* and *growth hormone*. These are useful only in situations of prolonged low blood
sugars, or fasts.

With this three-tiered protection from low BGs (stopping insulin
secretion, increasing glucagon and epinephrine, increasing cortisol and growth hormone), it is easy to understand that a healthy
person almost never experiences a low BG spontaneously.

Your Glucose Response with Diabetes

Now let's move on to you, since you now have diabetes. The first
point to make is that hypoglycemia is much less of a problem for
patients with type 2 diabetes than for patients with type 1. You got
a little bit of a break here. With type 2 diabetes, you are really only
likely to have a low BG (below 70) if you are taking insulin, or taking an oral medicine containing a sulfonylurea (we discuss these
pills in more detail in chapter 9). And even with these two medicines, low BGs are still quite unlikely for you, because as with type
2 diabetes, your pancreas is still secreting some insulin on its
own, and it can decrease this insulin when your BG goes low, putting on the brake.

On the other hand, the pancreas in patients with type 1 diabetes
has no insulin to secrete, and therefore patients cannot rely on this
first automatic brake. Patients with type 1 diabetes also lose their
glucagon response over time, and sometimes their epinephrine
response as well. These changes do not occur in patients with type

2 diabetes. In fact, several studies have shown that people with type 2 diabetes may release epinephrine at slightly higher glucose levels than people without diabetes, providing even a little more protection against hypoglycemia. One last extra protection present in patients with type 2 diabetes is their insulin resistance. Being resistant to insulin means that your BG will fall less dramatically in response to insulin—either your own or from an insulin injection. This relative insensitivity to insulin also gives your body's other responses more time to take effect.

What if you accidentally took an overdose of insulin? Would you die? This is actually a common question, but you can relax. You are not in any real danger unless you purposely take a massive overdose. Even if the worst-case scenario developed, and you passed out because of severe hypoglycemia, your body will recover, as it begins to increase its own glucose production, and you will wake up. After several hours, you should be back to your old self, without any permanent damage to your body. The real danger lies in receiving the too-large dose of insulin before getting into your car, or setting off on a swim across the lake, because you could pass out and harm yourself or others. This is why it's always important to check your BG before any potentially hazardous activities.

If you are taking insulin or a sulfonylurea, a more common form of everyday low BG might result from a missed meal or an unanticipated increase in physical activity. If you begin to notice the symptoms—fast heart rate, feeling sweaty, shaky, and hungry—you should check your BG immediately. Do not wait! And treat the low BG with a fast-acting carbohydrate if you are around 70 or less.

The best treatment is "pure" carbohydrate, meaning a sugary substance of about 15 grams. This could be 4 ounces of fruit juice, 5 to 7 Lifesavers or other hard candy, or 3 glucose tablets. Pure carbohydrate is important because it absorbs into your bloodstream immediately, raising your BG right away. A fattier type of sweet, chocolate for instance, contains sugar and is tasty, but the fat in it delays the absorption of the carbohydrate for up to several hours. Nutrition bars have the same problem, containing fat and protein that slow the absorption of the carbohydrate. If you don't have your glucose meter with you, you may not be able to tell whether your symptoms are caused by hypoglycemia or simply by overexertion, hunger, or anxiety. But to be on the safe side, it is reasonable to take some form of fast-acting carbohydrate if you feel funny. Naturally, you're better off when you have your meter on hand to check your BG to be sure.

In summary, low BG episodes are generally unpleasant. But you do not need to live in fear of them. Having type 2 diabetes, you are unlikely to experience them at all. If and when they do occur, you will be able to treat them quickly and appropriately. Try to turn a bad episode into a learning experience: think about why the low occurred, so that you can prevent a similar episode. This could mean a change in your glucose-related medication, or remembering to bring a small snack along when you're active, or have a later meal in an anticipation of a strenuous activity.

What You Should Know about High Blood Glucose

SINCE YOUR GLUCOSE numbers are so important in guiding your diabetes regimen, getting a high BG reading can seem very worrisome. However, we know that short-lived high BG levels cause no permanent damage to your body, even if you remain high for a few days. It is only when your A1c test is high—indicating high levels over weeks and months—that your chance of future complications increases. But even then, the real danger is only present when you have repeated A1c values that are above your goal.

Note: This does not mean that you should ignore high BG levels, but rather that you shouldn't be stressed over them in the short-term. It's the longer-term that matters here.

What happens if your BG remains high—above 200? The results are definitely undesirable. First, if you are in this range for several hours, your kidneys begin to filter the glucose into your bladder, and then also filter out extra water by osmosis, which results in increased urination, and increased thirst to replace your lost fluids. So you will be very thirsty and need to visit the bathroom often. If your BG is high for days or weeks, you may also experience blurry vision, as the lens in your eye changes shape slightly. This change is temporary, however, and is not related to any permanent eye damage.

When your BG is high for days, yeast infections are more likely, and other infections may not heal as well. High BGs over longer periods of time may also cause fatigue, and problems with concentration. This is not always the case, however, and many people with type 2 diabetes *seem* to feel perfectly comfortable at high BG levels. But this can cause a dangerous misperception; since they feel well, they may think that their diabetes is in good control.

It is very important to remember that the *only way* you can really tell if you are doing well is to know the results of your five diabetes tests. Feeling well is important, but it doesn't necessarily mean that your diabetes is under control. You don't want to ignore high BG over time. If your A1c is above your target, then your daily glucose results can give you information about the best way to change your regimen. If the high numbers seem more frequent than in the past, consider any lifestyle changes you've made that could account for the increases. If your trend of higher numbers on a daily basis persists, you can also consider repeating your A1c test sooner than usual to find out if this is truly having an effect on your overall glucose control (defined by the A1c).

Ups and Downs:
If I Wanted to Live on a Roller-Coaster, I'd Work at the Fair

MANY PEOPLE WITH diabetes are concerned about the ups and downs of their BG levels. Our advice: stop the madness. Stop the worry, that is. Certainly it can be frustrating to see your BGs fluctuate, often without an obvious explanation. This is where it's important to step back and consider your goals. Your primary goal is to live a long and healthy life with your diabetes. Remind your-self that your daily BG readings provide only part of your total risk picture. Remember also that your blood pressure may be even more important, and your lipids, microalbumin, and eye health status all contribute to reducing your chance of future problems. Now that you've established some perspective on your BGs, use your A1c as the most accurate indicator of your glucose-associated risk. As long as your A1c results are hitting your target, your BG values are actu-ally fine—with two important caveats:

The first caveat is that you are not experiencing bothersome low BGs. If you are having BG levels below 70 very frequently, you need to adjust your regimen, either by reducing your medication, or by taking in some extra fuel at critical times.

The second caveat is that your glucose control regimen should not be driving you or your family crazy. You should be able to find a compromise where you are eating foods you enjoy, and not feel-ing hungry or deprived.

If you are not having bothersome lows, and you are not going crazy with your glucose control regimen, then you are in great shape as long as your A1c is at or below your target. As we've pointed out repeatedly, the A1c tells you how your glucose control has fared over the last three months. Even if you had a few readings that you, or your family, or even medical personnel thought were too high, an on-target A1c tells you that they were not high long enough or often enough to be truly worrisome.

Would it be better to have your BG steady at 110 all of the time, with a good A1c result, compared to having the same A1c with BGs that are up and down? Some experts think so, but we believe there is no difference when it comes to the long-term effects of diabetes. When you have diabetes, it's pretty much inevitable that your BG will bounce up and down at times, often for reasons that aren't clear. None of this will affect your long-term health as long as your A1c is good. So find something else to worry about. And remember, less worry usually translates into better A1c results as well.

11 Heart and Blood Pressure Drugs:
What Can They Do for You?

I N CHAPTER 9, we talked about the growing number of medications available to help you control your blood glucose right now. Well, guess what? The medications we will discuss here may have an even greater impact on your future health.

The leading cause of death in patients with diabetes is heart disease. No need to feel singled out, however, since heart disease is also the leading cause of death in people without diabetes. Decrease your chance of heart disease and you are well on your way to leading a long and healthy life with diabetes. We've discussed the vital importance of keeping your blood pressure and lipids within target range. Essential steps to achieving these areas were physical activity and some attention to your diet. But what if these steps were not sufficient? Then what?

The next step would be to select one or more medications that can help you meet your goal. Let's be clear on why you would do this. Remember: you're not taking these medications because you have no other choice, or because your doctor told you to, or even because you "failed" to change your lifestyle appropriately. You are taking them because you know the importance of meeting your blood pressure and lipid goals, and you understand their effectiveness, when needed. In other words, you choose to take these medications as part of your own proactive efforts to live a long and healthy life.

Selecting the Right Medication for You

IT WOULD BE nice if patients could understand enough about these medications and their appropriate use, to be able to choose the right drugs for themselves. But that's not realistic. So you will need to rely on your doctor for guidance in choosing your medications. However, you are the one with diabetes, and you need to be involved with the decision-making process. Having a good idea about the drug choices available to you when you consult with your doctor will obviously be quite helpful, as is a proactive attitude.

In fact, clinical research has shown that doctors are frequently not as diligent as they should be in helping patients meet their health goals. A recent survey of a large representative health maintenance organization showed that over 40 percent of patients were not managed aggressively enough for their LDL cholesterol, and over 30 percent were undertreated for blood pressure. Remember that the health goals discussed in this book are based on national standards, and large numbers of clinical studies, so while our approach may be novel, the necessity of reaching these goals is not novel; it is basic care, and care that you deserve.

To get an idea of what medications could be most helpful for you, start off by reviewing your Diabetes Health Account. Do you have health debts in the blood pressure or lipid area?

Although many of these medications are helpful in several areas, we'll start off by sorting them into blood pressure, lipid, and heart groups for clarity (keeping in mind, as you know by now, that anything helping your blood pressure or cholesterol will also help your heart).

• • •

NOTE: BE PREPARED for a lot of medical jargon in the descriptions here. Don't let the unfamiliar terms put you off from learning about these important medications.

Also: The lists of drug side effects provided in this chapter are not necessarily comprehensive. Check with your doctor if you need more information.

Blood Pressure Meds

ACEIs and ARBs

Angiotensin converting enzyme inhibitors (ACEIs) and *angiotensin receptor blockers* (ARBs) are some of the most common medications used in patients with diabetes. Their main effect is on the *renin-angiotensin system*, a physiologic pathway important in maintaining blood pressure. Angiotensin, a polypeptide (molecule) in the blood, is the major player here, directly acting on blood vessels to increase blood pressure.

Angiotensin is formed in the body from a substance called *angiotensinogen*, which is produced and released into the circulation mainly by your liver. Angiotensinogen has no effect on blood pressure, but can be converted by a special enzyme into *angiotensin*. Blocking this converting enzyme decreases the amount of angiotensin that is converted form angiotensinogen.

ACEIs perform this very important action. Since their introduction in the 1980s, they have been used in millions of patients with high blood pressure. Clinical studies have also shown that they can be helpful for patients with heart disease.

Angiotensin affects blood vessels through actions initiated after attaching to a receptor that is on the outside of the cells. Blocking this receptor also blocks the action of angiotensin. ARBs are what perform this function. Although ACEIs and ARBs work on the same physiologic pathway, their effects are additive.

Both of these classes of medication also have an important secondary effect, in protecting kidneys. These protective kidney effects are not due solely to the lowering of blood pressure, but to a direct effect of these medications on the kidney. In patients with elevated microalbumin, an early indicator of kidney changes, both ACEIs and ARBs can bring about decreases in microalbumin, and decreases in the chance of future kidney problems. Because of this beneficial protective effect on the kidneys, ACEIs and ARBs are the initial medications of choice in treating high blood pressure in individuals with diabetes.

ACEIs

At present, all available ACEIs work in a similar fashion, and differ mostly in their length of activity (most need only be taken once a day), and whether they are available in generic form, as indicated by an asterisk below.

User information

GENERIC NAME	TRADE NAME	DOSE (MG)	DOSES PER DAY
Benazepril*	Lotensin	2.5–80	once
Captopril*	Capoten	37.5–450 total per day	3 times
Enalapril*	Vasotec	5–40	twice
Fosinopril*	Monopril	10–80	once
Lisinopril*	Zestril, Prinivil	10–80	once
Moexipril*	Univasc	7.5–30	once
Perindopril	Aceon	4–16	once
Quinapril	Accupril	10–80	once
Ramipril	Altace	2.5–20	once
Trandolapril	Mavik	1–4	once

Common side effects

The most common side effect of the ACEIs is a dry cough, which is unrelated to any changes in your throat or lungs. Sometimes switching to a different ACEI will relieve the side effect, but more commonly you will need to switch to an ARB.

ARBs

The ARBs presently available are listed below. At this time, none are available in generic form.

User information

GENERIC NAME	TRADE NAME	DOSE (MG)	DOSES PER DAY
Candesartan	Atacand	8–32 total per day	1–2 times
Eprosartan	Teveten	400–800 total per day	1–2 times
Irbesartan	Avapro	75–300	once
Losartan	Cozaar	25–100 total per day	1–2 times
Olmesartan	Benicar	20–40	once
Telmesartan	Micardis	20–80	once
Valsartan	Diovan	80–320	once

Common side effects

The ARBs rarely have side effects, but dizziness and headache sometimes occur.

Calcium Channel Blockers, Beta Blockers, and Diuretics

Although ACEIs and ARBs are almost always the first line medications used to control blood pressure, people with type 2 diabetes often need additional medications to meet their blood pressure goals, especially as their number of years with diabetes increases. Calcium channel blockers, beta blockers, and diuretics are the most common medications added. Each of these three different classes of medication reduces blood pressure by a pathway different from each other, and different from ACEIs and ARBs.

Why would you turn to these additional drugs? If you haven't reached your blood pressure goal with your current combination of physical activity, food changes, relaxation, and an ACEI and/or ARB, then you may need additional help. These medications are often used as second or third additions to your existing blood pressure medications.

Again, this does not mean that you have in any way "failed." Keep in mind that the insulin resistance at the genetic basis of type 2 diabetes is associated with high blood pressure that is slightly more resistant to treatment. That is, studies have shown that people with type 2 diabetes and high blood pressure will generally need more medication to control their blood pressure than do nondiabetic patients with high blood pressure. These same studies show that the beneficial effect of lowering the blood pressure is the same regardless of how many, or how few, medications are needed.

Your goal is not to take fewer medications, nor more medications, nor to compare your medications to other individuals. Your goal is to keep your blood pressure in a safe range by whatever means are necessary. The first approaches are always lifestyle modifications, including exercise, specific food changes, and stress reduction. If you've made all of the lifestyle changes that are practical and still need more help, then you need to turn to these very effective, very useful medications.

Calcium Channel Blockers

The *calcium channel* is a cell membrane transport system; blocking it can decrease high blood pressure. *Calcium channel blockers* are also used in patients with cardiac disease.

As before, those medications marked with an asterisk (*) are available in generic form; and those marked with pound sign (#) are available in extended-release once-a-day tablet form.

User information

GENERIC NAME	TRADE NAME	DOSE (MG)	DOSES PER DAY
Amlodipine	Norvasc	5–10	once
Diltiazem*#	Cardizem, Cartia, Tiazac, Dilacor	120–360 total per day	4 times
Felodipine*	Plendil	2.5–10	once
Isradipine#	Dynacirc	5–10	twice
Nicardipine*	Cardene	60–120 total per day	3 times
Nifedipine*#	Procardia, Adalat	30–180 total per day	3 times
Verapamil*#	Calan, Tiazac	120–360 total per day	3 times

Common side effects

These medications can sometimes cause fluid retention, and occasionally changes in the rhythm of the heart.

Beta Blockers

Beta blockers control blood pressure partly by slowing the contractions of the heart and decreasing your pulse. For people who've suffered a heart attack, they're effective in reducing the chance of a second heart attack. The best type of beta blockers for type 2 diabetes, listed here, are a type called *beta-1 selective antagonists*, which specifically act on the cells you need treated. Avoid nonselective beta blockers, which can have some negative effects on your glucose control.

User information

GENERIC NAME	TRADE NAME	DOSE (MG)	DOSES PER DAY
atenolol*	Tenormin	50–100	Once
metoprolol*	Toprol XL, Lopressor	50–100	Once

Side effects

An uncommon side effect of beta blockers is depression or fatigue.

Diuretics

Diuretics are the oldest class of blood pressure medicines. They work by reducing the amount of sodium in your blood, and also by mildly reducing your *intravascular volume*, which is the fluid present in your blood and other tissues. These medications are often called fluid, or water, pills.

User information

GENERIC NAME	TRADE NAME	DOSE (MG)	DOSES PER DAY
Hydrochlorothiazide*	HydroDiuril, Esidrix, Oretic	12.5–25	Once
Chlorthalidone*	none	12.5–25	Once

Common side effects

Diuretics can cause an increase in urination, in both frequency and amount, although this is less likely with the lower doses used to control blood pressure. They can also cause a decrease in your potassium level, so this should be checked periodically.

IN ADDITION TO these four main classes of blood pressure medicines, there a number of others: alpha blockers, aldosterone blockers, hydralazine, and more, giving you quite an array of tools that can be added to your lifestyle efforts. For this reason, your blood pressure counts as the risk factor that can be most directly controlled.

Lipid "Fat Busters"

NOW THAT YOU have your blood pressure under control, what about your lipids? Let's take them in this order: LDL cholesterol, triglycerides, and HDL cholesterol. Although we're talking about medications here, remember that exercise, and a shift to healthier types of fat in your diet, can decrease your LDL as well as increase your HDL cholesterol.

However, if these lifestyle changes are not sufficient, you are left with only two choices: change your genes, or add a medication. And since changing your genes is not presently an option, you're left with medications. One advantage you have is that millions of people have already made this choice, and you are able to use their experience and results to guide your own choices.

Statins

By far the most common choice of lipid medications is a *statin*. These medications, highly used and highly advertised, are also highly effective. Although pharmaceutical ads on television are often misleading (*Why* would you sit outside in a bathtub gazing at the horizon? And does the drug Cialis make it easier or harder to do this?), in the case of the statins the text of the ads (if not their visual imagery) are mainly accurate. Multiple clinical trials have shown their effectiveness, in both men and women, in lowering LDL cholesterol and reducing heart attacks. Some recent studies have shown that the reduction in heart attacks exceeds the benefits of lowering LDL alone. Statins seem to reduce inflammation, and are also able to reduce elevated *C-reactive protein* (CRP) levels, another cardiac risk factor. Moreover, smaller studies have shown possible beneficial effects on increasing bone density, and decreasing the chance of Alzheimer's disease. So statins seem to have health benefits on a number of fronts.

Of course, some people prefer "natural" supplements instead of pharmaceutical medications. If you are a member of this group, you will be interested to know that statins were discovered in Japan, where researchers were testing the health benefits of fungal broths. What could be more natural than a nice fungal broth? Something like mushroom soup with health benefits?

User information

If you need a statin, a variety are available, with little discernible difference in their effects. Generic kinds are asterisked.

GENERIC NAME	TRADE NAME	DOSE (MG)	DOSES PER DAY
atorvastatin	Lipitor	10–80	once
fluvastatin	Lescol	20–80	once
lovastatin*	Mevacor, Altoprev	20–80	once
pravastatin*	Pravachol	10–80	once
rosuvastatin	Crestor	10–40	once
simvastatin	Zocor	20–80	once

Common side effects

Side effects are actually quite uncommon. The most likely is an elevation in liver enzyme tests, such as the ALT and AST. These should be checked before starting a statin, and then again six to eight weeks later. If your levels remain in the normal range, checking once or twice a year is sufficient. If there are elevations, the dose can be lowered, or another statin tried. Cases of permanent liver damage are extraordinarily rare, and do not seem more likely in patients taking statins than in other people.

An even less common side effect is overall severe muscle aching. If this occurs, the statin should be stopped, and you should see a doctor immediately to have blood tests run to check whether the symptoms are associated with the medication.

In the case of mild muscle aches, you can try a brief trial of stopping the statin to see if it changes your symptoms, and then consulting with your doctor about further steps.

IF YOU ARE unable to take a statin because of its side effects, or if your LDL remains high after maximizing your dosage, there is a separate drug you can try, called *ezetimibe* (trade name Zetia). This drug works on a different pathway to lower LDL cholesterol. Its effects are additive to the statins, but it is also effective when taken alone, although not as potent. It comes in a single 10 mg dose, or is also available as a combination with the statin medication simvastatin (the combination marketed under the trade name Vytorin).

Bile Acid Sequestrants, Fibrates, and Nicotinic Acid

Although statins are the most frequently used medications for lipid management, several other classes of drugs can be very helpful yet are often underutilized. These are called *bile acid sequestrants*, *fibrates*, and *nicotinic acid*.

Bile Acid Sequestrants

Bile acid sequestrants have a primary effect on lowering LDL cholesterol, although they are not quite as potent as statins. They have a more beneficial effect than statins on your HDL, usually increasing this healthy cholesterol. As their name suggests, they act by binding to the bile acids in your intestine. These bile acids are involved in transporting cholesterol in your system, so when their number is effectively reduced (by binding them to bile acid sequestrants), your LDL cholesterol is reduced, and your HDL cholesterol increased. Because they work on a different pathway than the statins, their LDL lowering effect is complementary to the effect of the statins. The sequestrants are not absorbed from your intestines, so they never enter your blood stream, and thus have no side effects outside of your bowels. However, they do have some side effects in your bowels, as described below. The newest addition to this class, *colesevelam*, has fewer side effects and is usually better tolerated.

User information

GENERIC NAME	TRADE NAME	DOSE	DOSES PER DAY
Colesevelam	Welchol	3.8 total per day	Once or twice
Colestipol	Colestid	10 total per day	Once or twice
Cholestyramine*	Questran	8 total per day	Once or twice

Common side effects

Since these medications are not absorbed into your body, they have only local side effects in your bowels, which may include constipation, nausea, heartburn, and gas. These are less likely with colesevelam. They have no hidden side effects; if you feel okay, there is nothing else that you or your doctors need to check. These drugs work very well in combination with the statins, and are generally underutilized.

Fibrates

Fibrates act on parts of the same intracellular PPAR system that are affected by glucose-lowering thiazolidinediones, although fibrates have no effect on your blood glucose. Like bile acid sequestrants, their effect is additive to that of statins. Although they can lower LDL cholesterol, their major effect is in lowering triglycerides and increasing HDL cholesterol. This means they are a good fit for people with metabolic syndrome, as high triglycerides and low HDL cholesterol are primary components of that syndrome. When used with statins, these drugs can increase the chance of *myopathy*, or muscle aching. However, this side effect is uncommon.

User information

GENERIC NAME	TRADE NAME	DOSE (MG)	DOSES PER DAY
Fenofibrate	Tricor	160	Once
Gemfibrozil*	Lopid	1,200 total per day	Twice

Common side effects

These medications may cause an elevation of liver enzymes or muscle enzymes similar to that of statins, and, when used with a statin, the chance of these side effects is slightly higher.

Nicotinic Acid

Nicotinic acid, or niacin, is a vitamin B_3 derivative that lowers LDL and triglycerides, and has the largest effect on increasing HDL cholesterol of any medication. Nicotinic acid is available over the counter without a prescription, and is usually taken three times a day. Usage is sometimes limited by a common skin side effect of flushing and itching. Taking this medication more gradually helps decrease these side effects, therefore two longer-lasting preparations are available: a sustained-release form, absorbed over 12 to 24 hours, and an extended-release form, absorbed over 8 hours.

User information

GENERIC NAME	TRADE NAME	DOSE (MG)	DOSES PER DAY
Nicotinic acid (niacin)*	None, available without a prescription	Start slowly, work up to 2 grams/day	Three
Nicotinic acid—extended release	Niaspan	Start slowly, work up to 2 grams/day	Once
Nicotinic acid—sustained release	Niacor, Slo-niacin	Start slowly, work up to 2 grams/day	Once

Common side effects

Flushing and itching can occur with all three forms, but are less common with the longer-release forms. These symptoms can decrease over time, and may also be decreased by taking an aspirin before the nicotinic acid. The extended release form has been associated with liver side effects, more than the other two forms, and it should probably be avoided. The sustained-release form Niaspan is currently preferred, because it causes fewer side effects than the others. Early studies of nicotinic acid use showed mild elevations in blood glucose, so in the past it was often avoided in patients with diabetes. However, for most people with diabetes, the effect on blood glucose is minor, whereas the positive effect on HDL and triglycerides can be very beneficial.

Baby Aspirin—Not Just for Kids

FINALLY, WE CANNOT close this chapter without mentioning the effects of baby aspirin—for adults, that is. Low doses of aspirin, in the range of 81 mg—the amount contained in one baby aspirin—have been shown to decrease the chance of stroke and cardiovascular disease over time. This low dose is frequently given to patients without diabetes who have a risk, or history, of heart attacks or strokes. The current recommendations for people with diabetes is that anyone with type 2 who is over the age of thirty can benefit from a daily tablet of baby aspirin. Side effects of low-dose aspirin are quite uncommon, but include ringing in the ears and bleeding from your stomach or intestines. This sounds scary, but is extremely rare, so don't let it put you off the benefits of low-dose aspirin.

12 Diabetes Devices

THERE ARE A lot of gadgets associated with diabetes care. Some of them are essential, and others are personal choices, depending on how much you like gadgets and whether you are the type of patient who likes to be on the cutting edge of aggressive new treatments.

Meters and Lancets

IF YOU HAVE diabetes, there's no getting around glucose meters and lancets. They're part of your life now: essential tools for keeping yourself healthy. (See chapter 6 on why it's so important to use your meter.) You're going to be carrying these items with you virtually everywhere, so you want to find a metering system that you like, meaning you understand the features you need and you're comfortable using the device.

There are at least a dozen popular meters available now, and they all work pretty much the same way. They include some kind of lancing device, generally a sort of wand topped with a spring-operated needle (the *lancet*), which you'll need to replace periodically. The meter itself looks like a minicomputer that about fits in the palm of your hand. It has an LCD window for showing results, and a few buttons on its face. And you will need to carry at least one vial of the little strips you insert in the meter for gathering the blood sample each time you test. These components come packaged in a nice compact carrying case with pockets for extra lancets and your vial of test strips.

The various features of the monitors are mostly nonessential, subjective choices: you might prefer a larger meter because it's easier to hold, whereas another person might want a smaller, more portable model.

Here are some of the key features to consider when choosing your meter:

- Meter size
- Test sample (how much blood is needed to activate the test)
- Test time window (how long you have to get the blood on the strip)
- Length of test (how long it takes to get results)—look for five seconds or less
- Font size and lighting (how easy it is to read the results window)
- Meter memory options (some new models make this much easier to use)
- Alternate site testing (how easy is it to use the meter on forearms or thighs?)
- Integration (meter will communicate with a pump or a software program for results tracking)
- Test strip handling system (uses individual test strips or contains a disc allowing multiple tests)
- Test strip cost

The price of glucose meters ranges from about $30 to $120. These days, many meters are also available for free through your doctor or certified diabetes educator (CDE). It's the test strips that are expensive, and this is true in varying degrees for all brands. Be sure to check with your health insurance plan in advance to find out which test strips will be cheapest for you. This may be the deciding factor in your choice of meter. Especially if you do not have insurance, you'll want to compare the current cost of test strips, which can run anywhere from 40 cents to $1 or more per strip.

Popular meter brands

- Abbott (Precision Xtra, FreeStyle, FreeStyle Flash)— http://abbottdiabetescare.com/
- Accu-Check (Active, Advantage, Compact)— www.roche-diagnostics.com/products_services/ productfamily.html?productfamily=Accu-Chek
- Ascencia (Breeze, Contour, DEX2, Elite)— www.bayercarediabetes.com/prodServ/products/index.asp
- Home Diagnostics (TrueTrack, TrackEASE)— www.homediagnosticsinc.com/products.asp
- LifeScan OneTouch— www.lifescan.com/products/meters/
- Medisense Optium from Liberty Medical— www.libertymedical.com/d_glucose_meters.asp

Another new option is the Sidekick all-in-one disposable meter from Home Diagnostics, available in many retail/drugstores for about $32. It's a small vial of 50 test strips with a built-in meter on top, including a carrying case. This might be ideal for travel, or a backup in case you get caught somewhere without your meter. (For product details, see www.prestigesmartsystem.com/products-sidekick.asp.) Note that the Sidekick does *not* include a lancing device; the manufacturers assume you'll use one you already own. You can buy separate lancing devices at most drugstores for about $15 without a prescription.

Backups are imperative, because you never know when your meter might poop out on you, or you simply forget to bring it along.

Most people have at least two—one they keep at home and one they carry with them. It's also a great idea to keep an extra set of the batteries your meter requires, in your cupboard and/or your car.

IMPORTANT METER SHOPPING TIPS

- Especially if you don't have health insurance, look for glucose meters and in particular the test strips at large discount stores like Wal-Mart and Costco. You don't need a prescription to buy these items, and you can save a considerable amount of money by comparison-shopping.
- You don't have to use the lancing device that came with your meter, if you don't like it. For about $15, you can buy one separately, with the design and lancet needles of your choice.
- If you get a backup meter, make sure it uses the same test strips as your regular meter—otherwise you'll have to purchase an entire second set of expensive strips.

Lancing devices and the little needles they use—which come packaged with your meter—also vary in shape and size. Most newer lancing devices have a little gear that allows you to dial the depth of penetration. Most also include an optional clear plastic cap that is used for testing on sites other than your fingertips (usually forearm or thigh) for deeper penetration, permitting you to draw enough blood for the test.

Most lancet needles fit into almost any meter model. But they differ in the *gauge*, or width of the metal point that sticks your finger. The higher the gauge, the smaller the hole in your finger. A 30-gauge lancet makes a smaller hole than a 23-gauge lancet. Many people find that a 30-gauge lancet hurts less, too, but everyone's sensitivity is different. One potential drawback to using a higher-gauge lancet is that you may not get enough blood, so you may find yourself repeating fingersticks over and over. Not so nice.

Just keep in mind that the lancing device packaged with your meter may not be the best one for you. There are plenty of others to choose from. If you can't get enough blood or it hurts too much, ask your doctor or educator to let you try some samples from other models in their office, so that you don't waste money buying another device that you don't really like.

Continuous Glucose Monitors

A VERY NEW area of technology is *continuous glucose monitoring*. Rather than providing a one-time "snapshot" of your blood glucose at a single point in time—as today's meters do—new continuous monitors will deliver readings every few minutes around the clock, so you can watch the whole "movie."

The devices on the fast track to patients now are *subcutaneous*, meaning they're inserted under the skin via a tiny flexible probe, which is connected to a controller unit either via a small plastic tube, or wirelessly, using infrared technology. They measure your BG levels in the *interstitial fluid* (the fluid surrounding body cells) every 5 minutes and store the readings. The data can later be downloaded to a computer to produce detailed charts of your glucose levels throughout the day.

The major advantages of continuous monitors are:

- They provide information on your BG trends, so you can make adjustments in your regime (although at this time patients are still required to take fingerstick readings with a traditional meter before making decisions about insulin doses).
- There are safety guards. Alarms alert you to hypoglycemia (dangerously low blood glucose levels) or hyperglycemia (dangerously high blood glucose levels) the moment they hit.
- They enable you to have improved glucose control. Studies show that using a continuous monitor can make an

enormous difference for both type 1 and type 2 patients—
crucial for avoiding long-term diabetes complications.

But continuous monitors are still in the early stages, meaning that accuracy is still being studied. They actually require several daily calibrations with your regular glucose meter. In part for
this reason, they are still quite pricey and not yet covered by
most insurance plans. The two models approved by the FDA (for
BG trend-tracking only) and available to patients at publication
time are:

- MiniMed Guardian RT (also the Paradigm model,
  which is combined with a MiniMed insulin pump)—
  www.minimed.com/products/guardianrt
- DexCom STS (wireless and tubeless model)—
  www.dexcom.com

Insulin Pens

THESE DAYS, THERE are many more convenient ways to administer insulin than the traditional vial and syringe. Insulin pens are a
popular option because they're easy to use and carry, and virtually
pain-free—because they use tiny, disposable needles.

An insulin pen indeed resembles a large pen, one that uses an
inset insulin cartridge for the "ink." Some pens come prefilled with
insulin and are completely disposable; you throw the pen away
when you are through with it. Others are reusable; you just replace
the insulin cartridge whenever necessary. (Pens carry one type of
insulin only, therefore pens are not suitable for people who need
to mix insulins.) Dosing is very accurate, with some pens even
offering half-unit increments.

The pens administer rapid or short-acting (bolus) insulin used
to cover the carbohydrates eaten. The only exception is a new pen
from Aventis Pharmaceuticals recently introduced as an alternative

way to administer the company's long-acting (basal) insulin called Lantus. That pen is called OptiClick. More information can be found at www.opticlick.com.

In the United States, bolus insulin pen products are available from the following companies:

- Novo Nordisk (using their NovoLog insulin andEli Lilly insulin pens)—www.novonordisk.com/diabetes/public
- Eli Lilly (using their Humalog, regular, and NPH insulins)—www.lillydiabetes.com/product/insulin_pens.jsp
- BD Diabetes (pen needles)—www.bddiabetes.com/us/product/pen_needles.asp
- Aventis (Lantus pen)—http://en.sanofi-aventis.com/rd/portfolio/p_rd_portfolio_metabo.asp

Here are some of the key features to consider when shopping for an insulin pen:

- The brand and type of insulin the pen delivers
- The total amount of insulin that the pen holds when full
- The smallest and largest dose sizes that can be injected with the pen
- How finely the dose can be adjusted by the pen. For example, many pens offer doses in one-unit increments (1, 2, 3, etc.), whereas others offer only two-unit increments (2, 4, 6, etc.), and a few offer half-unit increments (1, 1½, 2, 2½, etc.).
- The styling and appearance of the pen and the material it's made from (plastic or metal)
- The size of the numbers on the pen's dose dial and whether they're magnified
- The amount of strength and dexterity required to operate the pen
- How you can correct a mistake if you dial the wrong dose into the pen

- The way the pen indicates whether or not there's enough insulin left remaining for your entire dose
- Whether the pen is disposable or reusable

Again, much of this is subjective choice. You'll want to find a pen that you can read and use easily. A great resource for further information on insulin pens is found at www.diabetesmonitor.com/pens.htm.

Pumps

AN INSULIN PUMP is a device about the size of a deck of cards or a pager, which can be worn on a belt or kept in a pocket. The pump connects to narrow, flexible plastic tubing that ends with a needle inserted just under the skin. The pump is set to automatically administer a steady trickle, or basal amount, of insulin continuously throughout the day. By pushing a button, you can release bolus doses of insulin (several units at a time) at meals, and whenever you feel your BG is too high.

Let us be clear: an insulin pump is *not* an artificial pancreas or a cure for diabetes.

Unlike a healthy pancreas, a pump cannot work automatically; it can't decide how much insulin you need or when you need it—which makes the person running it the most important part of the pump. You still need to use a glucose monitor to check your BG levels, plus you must count carbohydrates in order to calculate how much bolus insulin is needed, and then punch in the correct amount of insulin dose. You also still need to attend to other diabetes-related health matters independent of insulin.

For people who would otherwise need multiple injections throughout the day, however, the advantages to wearing an insulin pump are:

- It does away with syringes and multiple injections.

- It eliminates the need to carry loose diabetes supplies (other than a meter).
- It provides continuous basal insulin at very precise doses.
- You have more intense control: the pump can increase your insulin temporarily to cover times of illness, stress, or travel.
- You have more flexibility: when you eat meals or snack, dosing is as easy as a few button presses.
- It uses only short-acting insulin (no mixing or changing required).
- It has a single small, fine needle.

But there are also some lifestyle issues to consider:

- You need to check your BG more frequently: Pump users must be willing to check at least four times a day—to obtain the information necessary to make good dosing decisions.
- You may object to feeling tethered: some people are concerned about being "attached" to a device 24/7. This is probably the single largest obstacle most people face when considering pump therapy. Yet the overwhelming majority of people who initiate pump therapy never go back to injections.
- The pump can't be set once and forgotten: you will have to remove the pump every three days to plug in a fresh insulin cartridge, and change the site on your skin where the pump is replugged in. Some people have trouble with irritation, and/or infections at these sites.
- There are other mechanical difficulties: tubing can get kinked, or alarms malfunction, or the unit itself can fail (note that pump companies are very responsive about replacing failed units).
- The cost may be prohibitive: many insurance providers require exhaustive proof that the patient needs pump

therapy, plus deductibles apply. But more and more insurance providers are recognizing the advantages of pumps and therefore covering costs. Pump companies will often assist you in negotiating coverage.

There are a number of ingenious models of insulin pumps to choose from. While they all work in a similar manner, they differ in terms of programming options, battery types, infusion sets (the patch where the pump is attached to your skin), insulin reservoir styles, and manufacturer's warranties.

Here are some items to compare when searching for a pump:

- Size
- Weight
- Battery life
- Infusion sets (the needle-and-adhesive set that attaches to the body)
- Number of different basal rates available
- Basal range (largest and smallest doses possible)
- Obstruction alarm (does the pump let you know if there's some kind of clog?)
- Overdelivery alarm
- Near-empty alarm
- Reservoir size (total amount of insulin the pump can carry)
- Warranty
- Special features (additional software often provides extra memory, multiple program possibilities, carbohydrate calculators, etc.)

Leading companies offering insulin pumps in the United States include:

- Accu-Check Spirit—www.disetronic-usa.com
- Animas—www.animascorp.com

- Deltec Cozmo—www.cozmore.com
- Medtronic Minimed—www.minimed.com
- Nipro Amigo—www.niprodiabetes.com
- Insulet OmniPod—www.myomnipod.com (new tubeless model)

JET INJECTORS—ANOTHER, LESSER-KNOWN OPTION

JET INJECTORS ARE simple, handheld devices smaller than an average remote control unit. They release a tiny stream of insulin forced through the skin under high pressure. They've been around for years, but are still not widely used, mainly due to underpromotion and the notion that jet injectors are painful.

PROS:
- No needles are required.
- This device may benefit people with needle-phobia.
- No syringes = no sharps disposal.

CONS:
- Bruising is common.
- The injector may not be as painless as it appears.
- There are sterilization issues.
- The available models are expensive.
- Insurance coverage is often problematic.
- Insulin dosing may be less precise, and absorption can be inconsistent.

In the United States, jet injectors are available from:
- Medi-Ject Corporation—www.mediject.com
- Bioject Corporation (formerly Vitajet)—www.bioject.com

Supply Carrying Cases

ONE OF THE biggest hassles of having diabetes, especially if you're on insulin, is the logistics of carrying all your supplies around with you everywhere. As noted, glucose meters generally come with their own special carrying case, with pockets for your test strips, lancets, and log book. But there is an ever-growing array of day organizers and travel bags to choose from, for carrying "loose medications" including pills, vials and syringes, and glucose tablets or hard candies, such as Lifesavers, to treat lows (necessary *only* if you are on insulin or a sulfonylurea, which can cause hypoglycemia). These specialized diabetes carrying cases are so prevalent, in fact, that you can now purchase them at Amazon.com.

What you need to think about is how elaborate you want the case to be. A small eyeglass-case-size model is probably fine for keeping a few extra supplies in your car or at work. But if you're traveling, you may need a cooling system to keep your insulin fresh, and space for up to two weeks' worth of supplies.

Some things to consider when shopping for cases:

- **Material**—leather or heavy-duty polyester with padding? Is your case a fashion statement or more of a rugged "cooler" to protect your gear?
- **Robustness**—will the case get tossed around during travel or sports? If so, look for thick insulation.
- **Number of nooks and pockets**—lots of little spaces may be confusing for you. Will you waste too much time digging through your case looking for what you need?
- **Size**—does the bag hold supplies for one week? Two weeks? A month? Or is it too big?
- **Integration**—some bags are made to look like, and even double for, a woman's purse or a teenager's backpack, for example. Do you want to combine the items you customarily carry, or keep your diabetes gear separate?

There are too many models for us to list them all here. So we're offering a rundown of some very popular designs, along with some good Web sites for diabetes carrying-case shopping:

- **MEDPort organizers** (www.medportllc.com)—a variety of designs, including the Daily Organizer, with a refreezable ice pack to keep insulin cool, and a temperature monitor to make sure the insulin remains at the proper temperature. A separate compartment keeps a monitor at room temperature.
- **Frio cooling system** (www.friouk.biz/us)—convenient cooling system that works using only water. No freezing or melting ice involved. Maintains a constant temperature for up to 45 hours. Cases are like padded envelopes in various shapes and sizes.
- **Glucokit** (www.diabetesincontrol.com/issue195/glucokit. shtml)—helps users integrate meters and accessories into a pocket-size package.
- **Desang Kitbags** (www.desang.net)—looking like yuppie planners, these are specially designed to carry vials, syringes, lancets, etc., in a sleek bag that fits neatly inside a purse or briefcase.
- **Diabetes 1 Bag** (www.diabetes1bag.com)—pretty, roomy tote bags designed to conveniently carry diabetes supplies while providing ample space for the normal contents of a purse.
- **aDorn Designs handbag** (www.adorndesigns.com)—small, stylish and neat handbags specially designed for diabetes supplies, including a water-tight ice compartment.

Specialized shopping sites include:

- www.diabetesmall.net
- www.diabetesandtravel.com
- www.insulincase.com
- www.medicool.com/diabetes
- www.professionalcase.com

Logging Software

IF YOU TEST your BG multiple times a day, diabetes management software offers a great way to track and analyze all of the data your glucose meter is gathering. Although your handwritten notes in a logbook are good for immediate data, they aren't very useful for viewing a week's worth of data or more. The software, on the other hand, lets you easily create reports and graphs to help you understand the trends or patterns in your blood glucose.

Most manufacturers of glucose meters offer software companions to the meter, along with a data cable for connecting your meter to a personal computer, so you can download the data. This information can be printed, e-mailed, and faxed. So sharing your data with your doctor becomes a simple task.

Many glucose meter companies are also teaming up with insulin pump manufacturers so that the meter's software can share data with the pump's tracking software. This gives patients an enormous amount of data they can use to spot problems in their diabetes regimen, and help improve their BG control.

Additionally, there are a number of independent software programs for diabetes management that allow you to input your BG and A1c results, insulin doses, carbohydrates and/or exercise for detailed tracking of your own regimen. These come in several different forms. Some are Web-based programs that you can use online for free. Some are Windows PC software programs that you can purchase. A few of these are made specifically for calculating insulin doses.

A great overview of various diabetes software programs is available at www.mendosa.com/software.htm.

Insulin Inhalers

THE VERY FIRST inhaled insulin, called Exubera, was approved by the FDA in February 2006. At least three other companies are working on competing products that should be available within the next few years. The whole notion of inhalable insulin is still very new, and some important outstanding issues remain: Will dosing be precise enough? What will the long-term effects be on patients' lungs?

Nevertheless, the prospect of painlessly breathing in insulin is quite exciting. The delivery devices are like asthma inhalers, although they differ from each other quite a bit in size and design.

Exubera, from Pfizer Inc.
(co-developed with Nektar Therapeutics)

Exubera is a mealtime bolus insulin in powdered form that you take no more than ten minutes before eating. You insert a capsule of the insulin into the Exubera inhaler, pump the handle, and press a button. The insulin is released from the capsule and forms a cloud in the inhaler, which you inhale by drawing a regular breath through your mouth.

The inhaler requires no batteries or electricity, weighs about 4 ounces, and is about the size of a large eyeglass case when closed. At publication time, Pfizer had not yet released the cost of Exubera or details on coverage by insurance plans. However, the *Chicago Tribune* reported in February 2006 that Exubera is expected to carry a price tag of $4 per day in the United States, or three to four times the average daily cost of injected insulin.

Other products still in the testing phase:

TechnoSphere, from Mannkind Corp.

This unique powder-form insulin is inhaled into the deep lung using the company's proprietary MedTone inhaler, a little purple device that fits into the palm of your hand. TechnoSphere is also absorbed rapidly into the bloodstream, for improved BG control. The inhaler appears to be the smallest and most handy of the group.

The Eli Lilly/Alkermes version, called AIR Insulin.

The inhaler device is roughly the size of a large marker, smaller and sleeker and apparently easier to use than the Exubera device. Experts report that it looks extremely promising, as it has not exhibited even the minimal effects on lung dysfunction as had Exubera had in early studies.

The Novo Nordisk/Aradigm version, called AERx.

This uses a liquefied version of insulin, delivered via a larger, battery-powered inhaler device about the size of a paperback book. AERx can deliver more minutely metered doses, and the device also keeps a dosing log, two potential advantages for many patients. But the liquid formulation of AERx requires it to be refrigerated— a significant drawback versus the powdered forumulas that don't require temperature control. And the delivery device is quite bulky compared to competitors'.

THE MAJOR CONCERN with all of these new inhaled insulins is their effect on the workings of your lungs, your *pulmonary function*. So far, clinical studies do show that a small number of patients had some decrease in pulmonary function over several years of using the inhaled insulin, but these changes may be reversible. However, the effects of inhaling insulin over many years are not yet known. Current recommendations for use exclude anyone who has smoked within the last six months, or with other pulmonary concerns. And right now, anyone using the inhaled insulin is required to take formal lung tests periodically. Insulin dosing with the inhaled version is also different, because the inhaler devices provide a more limited range of insulin units than do other insulin-delivery methods.

PART 3

Under
the Hood

13 What Is Type 2 Diabetes?

Type 2 Diabetes = Insulin Resistance + Insulin Deficiency

DIABETES MELLITUS, OR "sweet urine," has been with us for thousands of years. Simply put, diabetes occurs when the level of sugar, or glucose, in the blood is too high.

In general, diabetes is divided into two types, 1 and 2, that together account for about 98 percent of all diabetes. (Diabetes in pregnancy, unusual types of genetic diabetes, and diabetes associated with other diseases, account for the rest.) Type 2 diabetes is one of the fastest-growing diseases in the world, and this growth has prompted a huge abundance of news headlines and articles. However, there is nothing new about type 2 diabetes. It is the most common type of diabetes, making up 90 percent of cases in both the United States and the rest of the world.

How the Disease Comes On

WHEN THE LEVELS of glucose are very high, in the 200s or more, a number of immediate symptoms can occur. The excess glucose in the blood is filtered out by the kidneys, increasing the concentration of glucose in the urine—resulting in the "sweet urine" that accounted for the Latin name. This increase in glucose draws in extra water, increasing urine volume and frequency, which in turn causes dehydration and increased thirst. This generally causes people to radically increase their fluid intake. In addition to excess urination, these very high glucose values can result in fatigue, blurry vision, bladder and vaginal infections, and more.

However, if the glucose is lowered somewhat, to below 250 for most of the time, these immediate symptoms will fade, and the individual may feel quite well. But if their BGs remain too high, indicated by an A1c level that remains above target, they will be increasing their risk for long-term complications later. It is these long-term complications—heart disease, stroke, amputations, eye and kidney problems—that are the major health risk. Feeling fine is important, but with diabetes, it is essential to know where you stand with regards to long-term diabetes "risk indicators": the A1c test, blood pressure, lipids, microalbumin, and eye status. Feeling fine now doesn't mean that you *are* fine.

Understanding the Science Behind It

TYPE 2 DIABETES results from two physiologic changes in our bodies: *insulin resistance* and *impaired insulin secretion*. The first factor is a resistance to the effects of insulin. The second is simply a lack of enough insulin to do the job. Insulin is a hormone, a protein secreted into the blood by specialized islet cells in the pancreas (a small organ behind the stomach that produces important enzymes and hormones). Once insulin is present in the blood, it serves as a key that unlocks a unique insulin receptor on the surface of cells. When the insulin inserts into the receptor, a number of important metabolic activities are triggered inside the cell, including the increased transport of glucose into the cell. This passage of glucose into the cell provides energy for a number of cell activities (and energy for your body). This transport of glucose into the cell also has the important effect of removing excess glucose from the circulation, preventing the accumulation of high glucose in your blood. This process no longer works correctly in people with diabetes.

People with type 2 diabetes have a resistance to insulin, meaning their bodies produce and secrete insulin correctly, but that its effect is diminished. The insulin is less able to perform its glucose-reducing task after the insulin receptor is unlocked. A number of promising avenues of research are looking to identify the exact defects that make this happen, but, to date, no single flaw has been identified that is responsible for type 2 diabetes. It is most likely that type 2 diabetes is caused by a number of different things and that, in most individuals with diabetes, a number of genes will turn out to be involved.

However, insulin resistance by itself is not sufficient to cause diabetes, because we humans actually have the capacity to make much more insulin than we usually need. In fact, insulin resistance is not uncommon in the population, but most people with insulin resistance simply produce more insulin—enough to keep their BGs within the normal range. You can even lose 90 percent of your pancreas, and will still be able to make enough insulin to avoid high BGs and diabetes.

The bad news is that individuals with type 2 diabetes do not have this ability. Their bodies have lost the ability to make enough extra insulin to overcome their insulin resistance. Their insulin secretion may go up, so that they may make more insulin than someone without diabetes, but it's not sufficient to fully control their high BG levels. Hence their glucose levels remain higher than normal, and they have diabetes.

Note that levels of insulin resistance vary between individuals, and can also vary over time within the same individual. Insulin resistance is increased by inactivity, by eating foods rich in carbohydrate, calories and fats, and to a lesser extent by carrying excess body weight. Note that these three factors are increasingly present in our modern lifestyle, accounting for the marked increase in the numbers of people developing type 2 diabetes.

The good news is that people with type 2 diabetes are usually able to reduce their insulin resistance through exercise, careful eating, and/or medication, often bringing down their BGs into the normal range. This doesn't mean they no longer have diabetes, but it does mean they are controlling their diabetes very successfully—and their chance of complications is practically null.

Why Does This Happen to People?

IF YOU HAVE type 2 diabetes, you have certainly wondered why you ended up developing it. Was it because you ate too carelessly or weigh too much? One thing that we do know is that you can't develop type 2 diabetes if you don't have the necessary genes. You can't make yourself develop type 2 diabetes. We know this because sometimes it seems that everyone in this country is trying to develop type 2 diabetes: they are exercising less, eating too much fast food, and weighing more! Yet only about 15 percent of people will ever succeed in developing type 2 diabetes. Everyone else will have normal BGs. (However, this unhealthy lifestyle does bring on increased risks for heart disease, stroke, and other serious health problems—if you value your overall health, you're not home free to overindulge.) So if you blame yourself for developing diabetes, don't. It was in your genes. Blame your parents. Or, if you have a good relationship with your parents, blame *their* parents.

You might ask why these genes for type 2 diabetes are so common. An attractive and likely hypothesis refers to type 2 diabetes genes as "thrifty genes." This stems from the concept that thousands of years ago, food was often scarce. If someone had genes that allowed them to store fat more efficiently, and to keep their BG a little higher when there was no food available, they would have a slight survival advantage. Study of some specific populations supports this theory.

Pacific Islanders, such as native Hawaiians, now have a high prevalence of obesity and type 2 diabetes, although these same natives were lean and healthy when first discovered by Western civilization. The original settlers of islands such as Hawaii were enterprising people who set off on long journeys, not knowing when or whether they would reach a destination. During these arduous trips, many died from starvation; those who survived until landfall were likely endowed with these "thrifty genes." They may have been a little fatter at the outset of the voyage, and were able to draw on this energy reserve when food became scarce. Likewise, the ability to keep their BG slightly higher during fasting may have provided them with more energy when it was most needed.

Now, however, native Hawaiians are surrounded by food rich in calories and fat, and work at jobs that require much less physical activity. These changes, and others like them around the world, account in part for the rapidly growing numbers of people developing type 2 diabetes. Over the next decades, China and India will overtake the Western world in the numbers of people with type 2 diabetes, as they steadily adapt our Western lifestyles of decreased activity and more processed calorie-rich food.

14

What Is Type 1 Diabetes?

Type 1 Diabetes = An Immune System Problem:
Destruction of Beta Cells

TYPE 1 DIABETES is a completely different disease than type 2 diabetes, in regard to the underlying causes and the genes involved. However, like type 2 diabetes, clinical type 1 diabetes is marked by high BGs, resulting in the same long-term health complications over time.

How the Disease Comes On

TYPE 1 DIABETES results from the slow destruction of the insulin-producing beta cells in the islets of the pancreas. This destruction is activated by the body's own immune system. The immune system is essential for survival; it protects us from bacteria and viruses, and is also part of our body's surveillance system against cancer. But in type 1 diabetes, this protective defense system gets turned around, and slowly destroys the body's healthy beta cells until so few are left that there is not enough insulin available to prevent high BG.

Although this destructive process is usually slow, and can take years before clinical diagnosis, the early symptoms of type 1 diabetes are often more dramatic than those in patients developing type 2. Excess urination and thirst can become extreme, and many patients lose weight rapidly—reducing down to skeletal proportions in a matter of weeks—because the body suddenly becomes unable to process the food coming in. Calories in the form of glucose are flowing out of the body through excessive urination, and the person is literally starving to death.

Once the diabetes is recognized, and insulin treatment started, patients may enter a "honeymoon" period, in which some of their beta cells are able to recover and make some insulin again. Sometimes the honeymoon can last for several years, during which some patients are even treated with oral diabetes medicines rather than insulin. These oral medications can be somewhat effective in the honeymoon period because they can increase the body's sensitivity to the low levels of insulin that are present, improving the BG further. However, the underlying disease process always progresses, and eventually the honeymoon ends and the patient will need insulin.

Type 1 diabetes has been traditionally referred to as Juvenile Diabetes, because it used to be, by far, and still is, the most common diabetes occurring in children. But this is changing. A number of studies now indicate that more new cases of type 1 diabetes occur in adults than in children. The average age of onset of type 1 diabetes is now in one's thirties. This data is well documented, but not well remembered; many adults with new onset type 1 diabetes are mistakenly diagnosed as having type 2, simply because they appear "too old to have juvenile diabetes." This confusion and tendency toward misdiagnosis was a major reason for changing the former name of "adult-onset diabetes" to "type 2 diabetes." Another reason is that more children are being diagnosed with type 2 diabetes as our society becomes less active and more exposed to unhealthy food choices. In fact, the increase in type 2 diabetes in children correlates well with consumption of two items: fast food and sugar-containing drinks such as soda and sports drinks. Type 1 diabetes, on the other hand, is never brought on by eating the wrong foods. It is strictly an autoimmune deficiency.

Understanding the Science Behind It

AGAIN, TYPE 1 and type 2 diabetes are quite different: the beta cell destruction underlying type 1 diabetes is not present in type 2, and there is no evidence of autoimmunity in type 2 diabetes. Conversely, in type 1 diabetes, there is no underlying insulin resistance (meaning insulin, when injected, can be readily employed by the body).

The autoimmunity in type 1 diabetes is very specific, and remains mostly a mystery to researchers. It is not directed against any other organs in the body, and not even against the pancreas itself, but only against the insulin-producing islet beta cells present in the pancreas. Even the nonbeta islet cells present there are not destroyed. Also, this autoimmunity does not inhibit your body's capacity to respond to infections, and does not increase the chance of any type of cancer. Nor is type 1 diabetes associated with other common autoimmune diseases such as lupus, multiple sclerosis, or rheumatoid arthritis.

However, there are some similar autoimmune diseases which do occur more often in people with type 1 diabetes than in the general population. The two most common are thyroid disease, in which the thyroid is either over- or underactive (in about 10 percent of patients), respectively called a *hyperthyroid* and *hypothyroid* condition; and *celiac disease* (in about 5 percent of patients).

Thyroid disease can be easily detected with common blood tests, and the treatments (usually oral medications) are very straightforward and successful.

Celiac disease is an inability to digest wheat/gluten, now called *gluten-sensitive enteropathy*, which can cause abdominal discomfort to varying degrees, sometimes with diarrhea and bloating.

Celiac disease results from sensitivity to a specific protein, *gliadin*, which is found in gluten, a kind of protein commonly found in wheat and many other grain products. The treatment is also straightforward but burdensome: a lifelong avoidance of gluten. Avoiding gluten will gradually improve the symptoms, and also stop any further damage to the intestines.

A few other autoimmune disorders also associated with type 1 diabetes are less common:

- **Idiopathic hypogonadism**—an odd name for poorly functioning ovaries or testes, which can result in fertility problems
- **Addison's disease**—which results in destruction of the adrenal cortex, the producer of steroid hormones, and necessitates lifelong replacement treatment with corticosteroids
- **Vitiligo**—a skin disorder consisting of splotchy areas that have a total loss of pigment
- **Pernicious anemia**—whereby a lack of B_{12} absorption results in anemia.

Although there is an increased chance of developing one of these if you have type 1 diabetes, the overall chances are very low, at 2 percent or less.

Why Does This Happen to People?

Is TYPE 1 diabetes a genetic disease, or it is caused by environmental factors? The answer to both is yes. At least four genes have been associated with type 1 diabetes, but we know that more genes are also involved, albeit with lesser impact than the currently identified genes. The strongest gene association is in something called the *major histocompatibility locus*, which controls immune response. However, these diabetes-associated genes are also fairly common in the general population, present in about 30 percent of individuals. This tells us that type 1 diabetes is multigenic, as compared with other genetic diseases which are caused by a single, "bad gene." Examples of the latter are Huntington's disease, cystic fibrosis, sickle cell anemia, and thallasemia (also known as Mediterranean, or Cooley's, anemia).

To develop type 1 diabetes, you need more than four rare genes, and perhaps more than one copy of some of them. Plus, studies show that even in people carrying all of these necessary genes, the disease only occurs about one-third of the time. Researchers say that what's not genetic is environmental, but we have no idea of which environmental factors are at work here. One theory is that a viral infection that weakens the body may kick in the destruction of beta cells. What we know for sure is that the two environmental factors important in type 2 diabetes, exercise and food choices, are not important in bringing on type 1. A combination of multiple genes and unknown environmental variables accounts for the fact that 85 percent of people who develop type 1 diabetes have no family history of the disease. For most patients, it just comes out of the blue—but not a nice blue. Researchers are hard at work studying these mysteries.

What researchers know about inheritance so far is this: The chances of a parent passing on type 1 diabetes to his/her child appears to be about 1 in 20, or a 5 percent chance. If the mother has diabetes, there is an even slightly lower chance of the child developing diabetes than if the father has it. If neither parent has diabetes, but one of their children develops it, then other children born to that couple will also have about a 5 percent chance of getting diabetes.

15 Prediabetes and Metabolic Syndrome

Knowing Is Half the Battle

BEFORE WE BEGIN a discussion of prediabetes and metabolic syndrome, there is one other metabolic state to discuss: unrecognized diabetes. There are currently millions of people in the United States and around the world who have full-blown diabetes but don't know it yet.

Unrecognized diabetes refers both to people with undiagnosed diabetes, and to those in whom the diagnosis was made but this diagnosis was poorly communicated or understood. This is quite different than prediabetes, which is a preliminary state before diabetes develops. Many people, particularly with type 2 diabetes, may have had diabetes for years before they learned of the diagnosis. In some of those cases, they may actually have been told about the diabetes, but in an indirect way that did not alert them to the seriousness of this disorder.

Believe it or not, "borderline diabetes," "a touch of sugar," and even "you should start watching what you eat" are phrases sometimes used by medical personnel in describing diabetes. Many patients hear these phrases, but do not connect them with having clinical diabetes, and consequently the disease often goes untreated. Occasionally such patients are given an oral medication such as metformin or glyburide, yet without being made to clearly understand that they actually do have diabetes, and therefore they are not aware that they need to start assessing their overall diabetes health status, or may suffer the consequences.

Prediabetes: Nipping Health Risks in the Bud

PREDIABETES, SIMPLY DEFINED, is a physical state before diabetes occurs, which we can now recognize based on modern medical techniques and knowledge. Note that the science is not yet sufficient to identify with total accuracy those people who will definitely develop type 2 diabetes. But recognizing and treating prediabetes helps us tremendously to get a leap on treating a type 2 form waiting in the wings.

What constitutes having prediabetes? The American Diabetes Association currently defines this condition as a person's having blood glucose values that are higher than normal, but lower than the numbers needed to diagnose clinical diabetes. Prediabetes can be detected using two different tests, revealing an "impaired fasting glucose" or an "impaired glucose tolerance." *Impaired fasting glucose* means that, when your blood is tested after fasting (usually in the morning after not eating for at least ten hours), your BG levels are greater than 100 but less than 126. *Impaired glucose tolerance* means that two hours after drinking a 75-gram glucose solution, your BG is over 140 but less than 200. This second test is also performed in the morning after fasting.

**Prediabetes = "fasting glucose" levels of
greater than 100 but less than 126 mg/DL**

To be diagnosed with diabetes (rather than prediabetes), your fasting glucose has to be 126 or higher, or your glucose tolerance test results are 200 or higher.

Most clinical studies show that about 40 percent of individuals with these higher-than-normal glucose results (either impaired fasting glucose or impaired glucose tolerance), will develop diabetes within four years. But this risk of developing diabetes can be dramatically reduced by obtainable changes in activity and diet.

This fact was clearly established in the landmark Diabetes Prevention Program (DPP), a major study completed in 2002 that followed more than 3,000 people with impaired glucose tolerance. Patients were randomly assigned to one of three groups: a medication group, a lifestyle group emphasizing exercise and weight loss, or a control group (which made no changes). Impressively, the lifestyle intervention group showed a 58 percent decrease in the number of people who developed diabetes. Interestingly, the average weight loss was not as much as the researchers had targeted (7 percent of body weight), and yet the lifestyle-change participants were able to maintain and often exceed their exercise goals.

What this study illustrated is that focusing on increasing your physical activity is very helpful to your health, even if it does not result in significant weight loss; and also that it is quite doable and maintainable as a practical goal. As you may be realizing, the treatments that are the building blocks for helping type 2 diabetes (physical activity and food changes) are the same treatments that are effective in preventing (or delaying) the development of type 2 diabetes in the first place.

Based on the increasing prevalence of diabetes with age, some authorities claim that *everyone* is prone to developing type 2 diabetes, if they live long enough. This is only speculation, aimed at calling attention to the growing prevalence of type 2 diabetes. In reality, there are still clear genetic markers that must be present for type 2 diabetes to occur. So one way of defining prediabetes is whether the genetic background exists in the individual. At present, researchers have not been able to pinpoint the major type 2 diabetes genes, so a family history of type 2 diabetes is the best present method for identifying whether you have a genetic risk. One close relative with type 2 diabetes could increase your chance by around 15 percent, and having two parents with the disease could increase your chance by 40 percent. These numbers are not well established, however, since lifestyle changes have a major impact on whether or when you will develop type 2 diabetes—even if you do have the genetic background.

Again, the main reason for all the publicity around prediabetes these days is that early intervention has proven to be highly effective in halting type 2 diabetes. By diagnosing prediabetes, many people have the chance to make lifestyle changes and/or take medications like metformin early on, and therefore prevent ever being diagnosed with full-blown diabetes.

Should You Worry about Metabolic Syndrome?

METABOLIC SYNDROME, SOMETIMES known as *Syndrome X*, has become a popular buzzword, both in the medical field and in consumer health marketing. Essentially, it's a collection of metabolic disorders, all resulting from insulin resistance, that when present together can lead to high risk of cardiovascular disease and premature death. But don't let media-hyped scare tactics frighten you.

As a person with diabetes, your better predictors of cardiovascular risk are your individual results for blood pressure, triglycerides, and HDL cholesterol—with even more information provided by your LDL cholesterol. Add to that your understanding of physical activity and food choices, and you have a much better indicator of your health risk than that provided by the presence or absence of metabolic syndrome.

Nevertheless, let's explore this syndrome a little more, so you have a thorough understanding of it. Although definitions vary, the most widely used current definition is the presence of at least three of the five metabolic abnormalities listed below:

1. Fasting glucose above 110 (above 126 is the criteria for overt diabetes).

2. High blood pressure (top number above 130 or the bottom number above 85).
3. Triglycerides above 150.
4. HDL cholesterol below 40 in men, and below 50 in women.
5. Large waist circumference (more than 40 inches in men, and more than 37 inches in women).

Researchers have confirmed that individuals having three or more of these indicators are more likely to develop cardiovascular disease, and are also more likely to develop diabetes. These associations are one of the reasons this syndrome is drawing so much attention, but the main reason is that more and more people are meeting the criteria for metabolic syndrome.

The syndrome was first recognized by Dr. Gerald Reaven at Stanford in the 1980s, when he reported that people with insulin resistance, but without diabetes, were prone to heart disease. It was later discovered that high triglycerides, low HDL cholesterol, and high blood pressure often accompanied the insulin resistance. This grouping is informative for researchers, as it points out that there may be similar underlying mechanisms behind these individual metabolic abnormalities.

What's important for you to keep in mind, however, is that blood pressure, HDL cholesterol, and triglycerides all have *independent effects* on your risk for cardiovascular disease. Having more than one of these factors out of range increases your risk further. Slightly higher than normal BG, or an increase in *intra-abdominal fat* (measured indirectly by waist circumference) also add to your cardiovascular risk.

So the presence or absence of metabolic syndrome does not seem to carry, by itself, any further cardiovascular risk in addition to the combined risks of the individual components. Also, note that heart disease is the leading cause of death in people *without diabetes*, as well as people with metabolic syndrome, prediabetes, and diabetes. Everyone needs to be knowledgeable about their blood pressure and lipids, interested in finding ways to increase their physical activity, and conscious of their food choices. Since you are reading this book, and many people without diabetes are not, you may be edging ahead of them in the race to a long and healthy life, despite your diabetes.

16 Will Your Children Get Diabetes?

You Can Help Your Children Stay Healthy

MOST PEOPLES' FIRST question about having diabetes is almost invariably "Why?" In regard to adults' developing type 2 diabetes, we answered this question in chapter 13. The important things to remember are that you didn't cause yourself to get diabetes; you unfortunately were dealt the "thrifty" genes that were helpful for humans in the past, but can be harmful in our present sedentary, fast-food society. The steps outlined in the first portion of this book are designed to guide you down the road to living well with your diabetes. We hope that you've found these steps helpful, and that you will join the many people who are outliving their diabetes. But you may still be wondering about your children's risk. How likely is it that they will develop diabetes, and is there anything you can do about it?

The answer is: there are specific actions that you and they can take to reduce their chances by helping them develop healthy living habits. The sooner these actions are taken, the more likely it is that they will be successful; "soon" means as soon as they are walking, if possible. Now that you have a thorough awareness of your own treatment needs, you are armed with you excellent resources for protecting your children.

> REMEMBER, WORRYING AND being overprotective of your children is not helpful. Instead, focus on proactive things you can do to help lower their risk of developing diabetes.

Start Early with Diet and Exercise

ALTHOUGH YOUR CHILDREN are more likely to avoid type 2 diabetes than they are to develop it, having a parent with type 2 makes them two to four times more likely to get it than the general population, and their risk could be as high as 20 percent. This number is too high to soothe any parent into complacency.

Note that this risk can be *greatly* reduced by two actions: (1) starting and maintaining regular physical activity, and (2) paying attention to the types of foods that are commonly consumed. In fact, if your children can start these habits at an early age and maintain them, they will not only decrease their chance of developing diabetes by 60 percent or more, they will also significantly decrease their risk of heart disease and other cardiovascular problems.

Research shows that people who were physically active as children are more likely to be active as adults. By "physical activity," we mean anything that moves their body through space: team sports, walking, running, biking, martial arts, gymnastics, dancing, hiking, roller blading, and so on. Physically helping around the house or yard counts, too. Encourage them to walk instead of driving them everywhere. Disengage them from long hours of stationary activities like television/video watching, electronic games and Internet use—during which kids are often snacking as well. Activity is especially important if your kids are already overweight or obese.

There is an even stronger relationship between eating healthier foods as a child and continuing to do so in adulthood. The biggest food risks among children have been shown to be fast foods (french fries are the leading culprit here) and drinks with glucose or other sugars added. The latter category includes many sports drinks, which are laden with sugar. Most children (and adults) do not need to increase their calorie intake by drinking calorie- and sugar-rich liquids. Even fruit juice needs to be drunk in moderation, because it's high in sugar and calories. Your children are better off eating a piece of fresh fruit. Extend what you've learned about following a healthy diet to preparing the same kinds of whole-grain, vegetable- and legume-rich, low-fat meals for them. Look for those fresh, nat-ural ingredients, rather than relying on processed, convenience, or fast foods. You can also become involved with other parents work-ing to eliminate unhealthy foods offered to children at schools in the lunchroom or available through on-site vending machines.

Developing healthy lifestyle habits early in life will greatly reduce your children's chance of developing diabetes. You yourself will probably be modeling these same healthy habits for your chil-dren; in helping yourself, you will also help them.

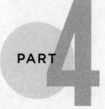

PART 4

Long-Term Living with Diabetes

17 Traveling with Diabetes

Enjoy Yourself!

DIABETES SHOULD NOT stop you from traveling and enjoying it. In fact, traveling really shouldn't be much different now than it was before you were diagnosed with diabetes, except that you'll need to pack any medications you take, along with some extras just in case. But fortunately, almost all modern medications are available in nearly any (Westernized) country these days—since diabetes, high blood pressure, high cholesterol and the like are common health problems the world over. These conditions are now part of life everywhere, so there's no need to stress out over medical supplies.

Please don't stress out over anything. Try to relax. Even if your BG is not where you want it to be while you're traveling—especially if you don't travel often—try to loosen up a little. Fretting will only make matters worse, and spoil your travel experience. This chapter will give you an overview of some proactive things you can do to assure a good time when taking your diabetes on the road.

Feet and Food

A FEW THINGS you will want to think about in advance are your feet and food, not necessarily in that order or in combination. Travel often includes increased walking (enjoyable and healthful) and new footwear (enjoyable and stylish). But this combination can sometimes lead to un-enjoyable blisters, so you should be thoughtful about adding new shoes to your mix. Your concerns about your feet are really no different than those of someone without diabetes, unless you have neuropathy in your feet, or a history of previous foot problems.

Be sensible about your footwear. Select high-quality shoes that are designed for walking. Don't wear a brand-new pair of shoes all day long on the first day or two, which tends to cause blisters from unfamiliar pressure points. In fact, it's a good idea to simply *change your shoes often*, so the support and pressure points on your feet are rotated. If you bought new shoes for your trip, try wearing them for a while before you leave, to break them in.

If you have neuropathy, avoid walking around barefoot, even if it's hot and the ground seems smooth and safe, or you are indoors. It's just too easy to injure your feet this way, or pick up tiny splinters that you don't notice until they cause real problems. Remember to pack a pair of slippers, rubber-soled soft booties, or flip-flops to wear in your hotel room, rather than going barefoot on an unfamiliar surface.

Finally, do take a few minutes to inspect your feet every day, perhaps before or after showering, just to make sure little injuries haven't occurred unnoticed. If you do get blisters, use disinfectant, soak your feet if you can, and be sure to swap out shoes so you're not wearing the same pair that caused the problem.

Food may be different when you're traveling. If you're anywhere in the United States, you can usually find something familiar to eat within five minutes (unless you're, say, backcountry hiking). But outside of this country, this is not necessarily so.

Also, the timing of meals will likely be "off" compared to what you're used to at home. In some countries, such as Spain, the dinner hour can be quite late; or while traveling your breakfast hours may be earlier than when you are accustomed to beginning your day at home.

Be prepared for these differences by carrying and eating snacks at regular intervals—and by keeping an open mind. The trip won't be as much fun for you (or your companions or hosts) if you're obsessed with set meal times or having only the foods you eat at home. Try to be flexible, knowing that you'll get back to your usual routine soon.

Planning Ahead

WHEREVER YOU TRAVEL, it never hurts to do a little planning ahead, because avoiding difficulties will make your trip that much better. Start by thinking about each destination individually: If you're going somewhere hot, will you need to purchase some sturdy sandals to keep your feet cool yet still protected? If you will be taking insulin, will you need to keep it cool? Remember that most insulins are good for a month out of the refrigerator, as long as the outside air temperature is not scorching hot. Check with your medical care team about your particular insulin. If you're going on long walks or hikes, do you have a good case for carrying snacks and supplies? If you are traveling to a foreign country, do you need to drink bottled water or perhaps even avoid eating fresh fruit or vegetables that may be tainted by local water? (You don't want a case of *turista*—or worse—on top of your everyday health considerations.)

Are you the kind of person who likes to make and follow lists? If so, you can start with the following prep list:

- Immunizations—top priority is not to get sick while you're away, so be sure find out what shots are required for where you are going, and get them on time (usually about a month in advance).

- Find out how long the flight will be and whether meals will be served. It's always a good idea to bring plenty of water and snacks, like granola bars, crackers or sandwiches. (Keep in mind that you can't take fresh produce into another country.) Also with tighter safety restrictions on international flights, you may need to check with your airline about whether you can bring pre-purchased food and drink on board with you.

- Bring a detailed list of medications—this will make your life so much easier in case you need replacements or refills. Ask your doctor to help you prepare a list of the exact medications you take, and their dosages. He or she can also look up overseas equivalents for you in case you need to replace or refill prescriptions on the road. (This applies to anyone taking medications, not just people with diabetes.) Always bring your medications in their original containers, or have copies of the prescriptions handy, so that security personnel can compare the description with the actual products.

- If you're going someplace very exotic (where prescription laws may be very different), you may want to write for a list of International Diabetes Federation groups: IDF, 1 rue Defaeqz, B-1000, Belgium, or visit www.idf.org. You can also get a list of English-speaking doctors at your destination (in case of an emergency) by contacting the American Consulate, American Express, or a medical school near you.

- Carry your medical insurance card, insurance emergency number, and/or medical travel insurance papers, if you have this kind of insurance. Also make sure you carry the name(s) of whom to contact in case of an emergency.

Especially if you're on insulin:

- Wearable diabetes identification—even if you don't tend to wear medical ID at home, you'll want to wear something recognizable, clearly showing the international medical symbol (Caduceus: a rod with two snakes entwined about it topped by a pair of wings) and the word *diabetes*.

- Plan for time zone changes. Talk to your medical providers in advance about how to adjust your individual insulin doses to account for time changes—or adjust the settings on your insulin pump, if necessary. With the new insulins in common use today, this is much easier than in the past.

- Be wary of hypoglycemia—people on insulin often "run low" in their BG levels while traveling, especially at night, because during the day they tend to walk more and eat less. Keep fast-acting carbs (candy, glucose tablets, gel, or sugary soft drinks) with you at all times, and be sure to bring along your glucose meter wherever you go.

- Pack two of everything—if you're taking insulin, the idea is to have a full set of supplies both in your suitcase and in your carry-on luggage. Your carry-on set can be a smaller quantity, but should be enough to keep you going for several days at least in case your luggage is lost. It will also be helpful for buying replacements if need be; you'll have samples on hand to show foreign pharmacists the pills, vials, or syringes you use.

- Ask your health-care team how to adjust your medications and meal times for a change in time zones, if necessary (and remember to adjust them again when you return home coming from the other direction).

SEE CHAPTER 9 for a list of the *names of generic equivalents* for common diabetes medications—which may be useful to have along when traveling.

Passing Security and Customs

OFFICIALLY, IN THE United States, you are supposed to notify air transport safety inspectors or personnel in advance that you'll be traveling with items used for treating diabetes. Unofficially, most people just show up at airport security with their supplies and all of the necessary paperwork. This includes a medical ID card, a letter from your doctor indicating that you have diabetes, a list of your prescriptions, and clear labels on each medication you're carrying (again, ideally in their original packaging).

As we mentioned, officials in most countries are already used to seeing diabetes medications and supplies, even syringes. But to avoid aggravation and delays, it's better to be prepared to show some proof of your condition, like your medical ID card or a letter from your doctor. This should be printed in clear, plain English on letterhead from the hospital or medical practice, so that foreign authorities can easily recognize the source.

If you do get stopped and questioned, the important thing is to be courteous and respectful. Don't get upset or argue with the officials, as that will only make them angry and/or suspicious, and prolong your delay. And once more, if you get stressed, your BG levels will likely rise, and you certainly won't be having as much fun.

Tips for Safety and Comfort

AGAIN, IF YOU like lists, here are some great additional travel tips from the National Diabetes Education Program (June 2005— www.ndep.nih.gov/diabetes):

- Keep your diabetes medications and emergency snacks with you at your seat—don't store them in the overhead bin.
- Don't be shy about telling the flight attendant that you have diabetes—especially if you are traveling alone. You

can often tell the airline ahead of time that you have diabetes and request your meal at a specific time. Although you may be able to pre-order a special diabetic or low-fat meal, carrying your own meal onboard is often a better bet.

- Always tell at least one person traveling with you about your diabetes.
- Just as for people without diabetes, moving around every hour or two (and taking breaks if you're driving) stimulates circulation and helps you stay comfortable

If you take insulin:

- Wait until the flight attendant is actually handing you your food before taking your insulin shot. Otherwise, an unexpected delay in the meal could lead to low blood glucose.
- If you plan to use the restroom for insulin injections, ask for an aisle seat for easier access.
- If you draw up your insulin dose from a vial, be careful not to inject air into the bottle (the air on your plane will probably be pressurized).
- Check your BG often. Changes in diet, activity, and time zones can affect your levels in unexpected ways.

YOU MAY NOT be able to leave your diabetes behind, but you can control it and have a relaxing, safe trip.

18

Healthy Feet and Mouth

Caring for Your Diabetic Feet

THIS BOOK FOCUSES on the core factors that you can control in determining your chance of future diabetes-related complications. Your A1c, blood pressure, lipid results, microalbumin, and eye exam provide the most important information for decreasing your risks. As we detailed in previous chapters, you can take specific actions to move these factors into a safer range.

There are also at least two other areas where you can make contributions to your diabetes health account: your feet and mouth.

You may have heard that foot problems are one of the major concerns for people with diabetes—with infections, slowly healing ulcers, and even amputations looming in the future. Similar to all the other complications we've discussed, foot complications (including amputations) are becoming less common among patients with diabetes. The major reason for this is the improvement in early detection and prevention of foot-related problems. Improved attention to blood pressure and lipids, along with a decrease in cigarette smoking among people with diabetes, have also contributed to this decrease.

Many people assume that foot complications stem from impaired circulation caused by atherosclerosis (or narrowing of the arteries), just as atherosclerosis in the heart and head can lead to heart attacks and strokes. This isn't actually the case. While circulation changes certainly contribute, a larger factor is neuropathy, which means injury to the nerves—in this case to the small sensory nerves in the feet. This injury is more likely to occur if your A1c remains high over time. It can cause numbness in your feet, often unnoticeable to you. The most sensitive indicator of this numbness is a decreased sense of vibration in your feet— something you are also unlikely to notice, but that your medical provider can easily check by testing your feet with a tuning fork (128 Hz or low C, for the musically inclined). You should be able to feel a "buzz" when the base of the struck fork touches each foot.

With decreased sensory input, your feet are more at risk for injury, partly because they are not constantly making the small microcorrections that you need to keep your balance, and to move the pressure points on your feet around. With this background of neuropathy, any decreases in blood flow to large or small vessels increases the chance of damage to your feet.

Smoking has a major negative impact here. Even if you're not worried about the other side effects of smoking—lung cancer, emphysema, strokes, and heart attacks—please be kind to your feet, and keep trying ways to stop smoking cigarettes.

If your Diabetes Health Account has a good balance, neuropathy and the consequential foot problems will be much less likely to occur. Keeping your A1c, blood pressure, and lipid results in a safe range are the most important factors.

There are a few more ways you can add some funds specifically to your Diabetes Foot Account. First, be sure that your health-care provider checks your feet regularly. These checks should include feeling your pulse in each foot, looking at the skin (including between your toes), and, again, checking sensation with some combination of simple devices: a tuning fork, a pin or pinwheel, and a small bendable fiber.

If you or your doctor notes any changes in sensation in your feet, or especially if your doctor identifies neuropathy or any other abnormalities, then you need to shift into "special foot protection" mode. This means taking extra care in choosing your footwear, not walking around with bare feet, and inspecting your feet yourself every day. What are you looking for? Any changes in the skin, a blister, a cut, or any signs of irritation. If you find such changes, watch them closely, and let your regular doctor or *podiatrist* (foot specialist) know immediately if they worsen, or if they don't improve within several days. This special attention to your feet will have a major impact on reducing your chance of future foot problems.

YOUR DIABETES FOOT CARE TO-DO LIST

- Wash your feet daily in lukewarm water, including between the toes. Dry them gently and moisturize well.
- Diabetes may cause you to sweat less, which can lead to cracked, dry skin. So when you trim your toenails, take care not to injure the surrounding skin, and use a clean tool that is specially made for toenails.
- If you have poor blood circulation in your legs or aren't able to see well enough to trim your nails, have your podiatrist do it for you.
- If you have neuropathy, wear moisture-resistant socks that do not have elastic in the cuffs, and well-fitting shoes with flexible soles made from crepe or foam rubber and soft leather tops that allow your feet to breathe.
- If you have neuropathy, avoid wearing slippers that are so padded on their soles that you have difficulty feeling where the floor is, which could lead to loss or balance and even falls.
- To prevent pressure sores on your feet, make sure your socks don't bunch or wrinkle inside your shoes.

Be sure to see your doctor if any sores on your feet don't start to heal in a few days.

If You Smoke . . .

WE MENTIONED SMOKING as being a particular risk factor for foot problems, not to mention being bad for your cardiovascular and pulmonary system. What should you do if you still smoke? The answer is obvious, of course, you need to stop, *right now*! Oh, right, you already knew that. You have tried to stop, of course, but haven't been totally successful. Or perhaps you are worried about failing, and haven't really tried. What can you do to stop smoking?

A quick survey of the medical literature shows more than 1,700 clinical studies, and over 12,000 articles covering programs to help people stop smoking. This clearly shows that stopping is not easy, but we do know that there are many methods that can help, and we know that fewer people with diabetes are smoking cigarettes now than in the past. Group sessions; medications such as Zyban; behavior modification approaches; and nicotine substitutes in any form—from patches to gum to nasal spray—have all been shown to help, though obviously not successful 100 percent of the time.

Still, studies confirm that people using these help methods are more successful than people who just decide to "tough it out" and throw away their cigarettes (although this also works for some). Most importantly, clinical studies have shown that the more often you try to stop, the more likely it is that your next try will be successful. This means whenever you try, even if you end up not quitting cigarettes, your next attempt is more likely to succeed. Your medical provider can discuss the different approaches, and help you find the Tobacco Control Program in your state to obtain a list of local programs and resources.

Cigarette smoking causes a constant drain on your Diabetes Health Account. Continuing to work toward quitting smoking is one of the single most important things you can do for your overall health.

Preventing Tooth and Gum Problems

ANOTHER AREA WHERE you can put away a few more diabetes health dollars is your mouth. (No, we don't mean stuffing the dollars in your mouth, but rather putting them toward good dental care.)

Most people associate dental problems with cavities, and it is true that preventing and treating cavities is important. High BGs may make cavities more likely to occur, although the evidence for this is not clear cut. However, diabetes most definitely increases your risk of gum disease and tooth loss, dry mouth, and a variety of infections. People with type 2 diabetes are particularly prone to gum infections, which cause inflammation that is damaging to your mouth, can in turn make your BG levels rise further, and is ultimately linked to increased risk for heart disease.

Here's how it happens: Day in and day out, high blood sugar caused by diabetes can contribute to the accumulation of **plaque**, an invisible film of bacteria, saliva, and food particles that covers your teeth. The bacteria feed on the sugars and starches in the foods and beverages you consume, and produce acids that damage the hard enamel coating of your teeth.

High BG levels give the bacteria a greater supply of food, allowing them to produce even more acid. The damage from this acid increases the possibility of tooth decay (what we commonly call cavities).

If you don't remove the plaque from your teeth with regular brushing and flossing, it hardens under your gumline into a substance called *tartar*. This tartar irritates the gums, causing a condition called **gingivitis**, which makes the gums tender, swollen, and red, so they may bleed when you brush your teeth. Fortunately, your dentist can prevent or treat gingivitis by removing tartar during a professional teeth cleaning.

However, untreated gingivitis can lead to a more serious condition called **periodontitis**, in which bacteria infect your gums and the bones around your teeth. This can cause your gums to pull away from your teeth and your teeth to loosen and even fall out.

Gingivitis and periodontitis are the most common oral complications of diabetes. If you have type 2 diabetes, you're three times more likely to develop gum disease than someone who doesn't have diabetes, in part because diabetes lowers your body's resistance to infections and slows your ability to heal.

The good news is that all of these problems can be quite effectively prevented. You just need regular removal of plaque by dental cleaning (about twice a year), routine tooth brushing and flossing, and maintaining a good A1c. As in most areas of diabetes self-care, maintaining good prevention is easier than trying to treat problems after they've already developed.

YOUR DIABETES MOUTH CARE TO-DO LIST

THE ILL EFFECTS of diabetes on your mouth can be prevented fairly easily, as long as you:

- Brush and floss your teeth at least twice a day.
- See your dentist and have regular teeth cleanings twice a year.
- Visit your dentist immediately if your gums bleed or look red or swollen.

19

Diabetes and Your State of Mind

THERE'S NO QUESTION that one of the hardest things about having diabetes is the emotional struggle. How do you stay upbeat if you feel like you are somehow being punished? Or when you simply feel overwhelmed by having a disease that requires so much attention?

Taking care of yourself with diabetes is indeed a "mental game," requiring you to learn to function comfortably on a number of levels:

- Personal (emotional)—fighting off negative thoughts
- Social—interacting with others in social situations without stress
- Behavioral—preventing yourself from doing things you wish you wouldn't, sometimes even self-destructive things

The first thing to know is that you are not alone in this. In fact, the psychological side of diabetes is now widely recognized and there are a growing number of programs dedicated to it specifically.

How Much Distress Is "Normal"?

EVEN THOUGH FEELING overwhelmed and negative is incredibly common among people with diabetes, traditionally there was no easy way to measure whether you were just experiencing the everyday frustrations, or whether you were genuinely distressed—and possibly in need of help.

New tools like the questionnaire "Living with Diabetes," reprinted with permission from the Behavioral Diabetes Institute (www.behavioraldiabetes.org), make it much easier for you to gauge where you stand with your level of distress.

LIVING WITH DIABETES: HOW DISTRESSED ARE YOU?

Feeling that diabetes is taking up too much of my mental and physical energy every day.

❑ 1—not at all
❑ 2—a little
❑ 3—more than a little
❑ 4—a moderate amount
❑ 5—more than a moderate amount
❑ 6—a great deal

Feeling that my doctor doesn't know enough about diabetes and diabetes care.

❑ 1—not at all
❑ 2—a little
❑ 3—more than a little
❑ 4—a moderate amount
❑ 5—more than a moderate amount
❑ 6—a great deal

Feeling angry, scared and/or depressed when I think about living with diabetes.

❏ 1—not at all
❏ 2—a little
❏ 3—more than a little
❏ 4—a moderate amount
❏ 5—more than a moderate amount
❏ 6—a great deal

Feeling that my doctor doesn't give me clear enough directions on how to manage my diabetes.

❏ 1—not at all
❏ 2—a little
❏ 3—more than a little
❏ 4—a moderate amount
❏ 5—more than a moderate amount
❏ 6—a great deal

Feeling that I am not testing my blood sugars frequently enough.

❏ 1—not at all
❏ 2—a little
❏ 3—more than a little
❏ 4—a moderate amount
❏ 5—more than a moderate amount
❏ 6—a great deal

Feeling that I am often failing with my diabetes regimen.

❏ 1—not at all
❏ 2—a little
❏ 3—more than a little
❏ 4—a moderate amount
❏ 5—more than a moderate amount
❏ 6—a great deal

Feeling that friends or family are not supportive enough of my self-care efforts (e.g., planning activities that conflict with my schedule, encouraging me to eat the "wrong" foods).
- ❏ 1—not at all
- ❏ 2—a little
- ❏ 3—more than a little
- ❏ 4—a moderate amount
- ❏ 5—more than a moderate amount
- ❏ 6—a great deal

Feeling that diabetes controls my life.
- ❏ 1—not at all
- ❏ 2—a little
- ❏ 3—more than a little
- ❏ 4—a moderate amount
- ❏ 5—more than a moderate amount
- ❏ 6—a great deal

Feeling that my doctor doesn't take my concerns seriously enough.
- ❏ 1—not at all
- ❏ 2—a little
- ❏ 3—more than a little
- ❏ 4—a moderate amount
- ❏ 5—more than a moderate amount
- ❏ 6—a great deal

Not feeling confident in my day-to-day ability to manage diabetes.
- ❏ 1—not at all
- ❏ 2—a little
- ❏ 3—more than a little
- ❏ 4—a moderate amount
- ❏ 5—more than a moderate amount
- ❏ 6—a great deal

Feeling that I will end up with serious long-term complications, no matter what I do.
- ❑ 1—not at all
- ❑ 2—a little
- ❑ 3—more than a little
- ❑ 4—a moderate amount
- ❑ 5—more than a moderate amount
- ❑ 6—a great deal

Feeling that I am not sticking closely enough to a good meal plan.
- ❑ 1—not at all
- ❑ 2—a little
- ❑ 3—more than a little
- ❑ 4—a moderate amount
- ❑ 5—more than a moderate amount
- ❑ 6—a great deal

Feeling that friends or family don't appreciate how difficult living with diabetes can be.
- ❑ 1—not at all
- ❑ 2—a little
- ❑ 3—more than a little
- ❑ 4—a moderate amount
- ❑ 5—more than a moderate amount
- ❑ 6—a great deal

Feeling overwhelmed by the demands of living with diabetes.
- ❑ 1—not at all
- ❑ 2—a little
- ❑ 3—more than a little
- ❑ 4—a moderate amount
- ❑ 5—more than a moderate amount
- ❑ 6—a great deal

Feeling that I don't have a doctor who I can see regularly about my diabetes.

☐ 1—not at all
☐ 2—a little
☐ 3—more than a little
☐ 4—a moderate amount
☐ 5—more than a moderate amount
☐ 6—a great deal

Not feeling motivated to keep up my diabetes self-management.

☐ 1—not at all
☐ 2—a little
☐ 3—more than a little
☐ 4—a moderate amount
☐ 5—more than a moderate amount
☐ 6—a great deal

Feeling that friends or family don't give me the emotional support that I would like.

☐ 1—not at all
☐ 2—a little
☐ 3—more than a little
☐ 4—a moderate amount
☐ 5—more than a moderate amount
☐ 6—a great deal

SCORE

0–20 Compared to most people, you have a relatively low level of diabetes distress. Congratulations. Still, there may be some specific issues about diabetes that are tough for you. Give special attention to anything that might help you feel even more comfortable and confident with your diabetes.

21–55 Compared to most people, you have an average level of diabetes distress. But that doesn't mean you should settle for this. The good news is that there is almost always ways to resolve stresses like the ones you are experiencing. Remember that you can't address all of these problems at once. The best bet is to talk to your health-care provider about what your next steps should be. If you don't have a good doctor or other health-care provider, your first task should be finding one that's right for you.

56–102 Compared to most people, you have a relatively high level of diabetes distress. The first step is realizing what your individual problems are, and accepting that you cannot address all of them at once. Instead, look for a professional health-care provider to help you tackle them one by one. Meanwhile, some ideas are presented in this chapter that may help steer you in the right direction.

Everyday Frustrations and What You Can Do about Them

WE HOPE YOU went through the diabetes distress questionnaire, because this tool can guide you just as the results on your Diabetes Health Account guided your actions toward reducing your health risks. Look over your responses to see if you uncovered some unrecognized areas of concern. What is really frustrating you the most? Your overall score also provides you with an idea of the level of distress, or frustration, that you are currently dealing with: high results mean that you will certainly benefit from having a professional help you find ways to alleviate your distress. This professional could be your primary doctor, a diabetes specialist or educator, or a therapist. Clinical studies have shown that if your level of diabetes distress is high, it's much harder to take the steps required to improve your health.

If your questionnaire results are moderate or low, you're probably just grappling with the nuisances of diabetes on a day-to-day basis. We talked a little about finding your own motivation in chapter 4. What it really boils down to is figuring out what matters to you in life: Are you pursuing a career that you enjoy? Are you in a satisfying relationship or hope to begin one? Do you have children already or desire them? Wish you could enjoy more recreational interests, additional schooling, volunteer work, or travel? Are you looking to spend more quality time with your grandchildren? Whatever it is, taking care of your health will help you pursue all the things that make you tick and make you happy.

A few important things can help offset general negative feelings about your diabetes:

- **Know the real odds.** This book is all about understanding your real odds for developing complications, and what you can do to improve those odds.
- **Fight fear with knowledge.** Learn about the powerful benefits of good diabetes care by working through the program in this book, talking to your doctor, and perhaps enrolling in a diabetes education program. Also, stay informed about the latest in diabetes care by subscribing to one of the popular diabetes magazines (such as *Diabetes Forecast*, *Diabetes Health*, and *Diabetes Self-Management*).
- **Stay in charge.** Remember that your own actions make the biggest difference to your health. As this book has shown you, you are not helpless. After all, it's not diabetes itself that typically causes serious problems, it's poorly controlled diabetes. With good care, you can live a long and healthy life.
- **Make sure your support team is really supportive.** If your doctor or other medical personnel tend to concentrate on discouraging news, shoot down your desires to try new treatments, or seems to take no genuine pleasure in your triumphs, maybe it's time to find another team. (See "Doctor Frustration" below for tips on how to handle this.)

Now let's look at some specific gripes shared by many patients across the country, and some suggestions of things you can do about them.

Feeling Lost and Alone

Isolation is perhaps the biggest grievance of people with diabetes. Most people lack a confidante who they feel really understands their experience living with this disease—often despite the many uncles, aunts, and cousins who may also have diabetes. And many people even have trouble finding a medical professional who they feel comfortable talking to.

In America in particular, we tend to have an "every man for himself" mentality, so being left alone with our troubles seems normal to us. But there's no underestimating the value of support community for everyone, from the newly diagnosed to the long-term patient feeling burned out.

What you can do

Get yourself out there in the diabetes community. You'll find that meeting other people with diabetes is actually a huge help to you personally, and also helps take the pressure off your family in helping you deal with your diabetes. Being able to toss out questions and ideas, and get support and empathy from others in your shoes is essential. This is where you'll get the best practical tips for everyday life with diabetes as well. It doesn't matter if you reach out to others in person or online. The point is to open up communications lines with others who share your concerns.

For in-person contact, finding local support groups, classes, and seminars is as usually simple as a quick Internet search, a scan through your local newspaper or phone book's community resources/events listings, or a call to your local hospital. Most of these programs are free or inexpensive, and offer a great way to mix with other people with diabetes and learn some ways to improve your health care at the same time. Many clinics and medical groups across the country now offer top-notch *personalized* programs as well, which allow you to talk over your biggest roadblocks with an educator or nutritionist.

For online contact, message boards, forums, and Web logs all allow you to connect with other people in your shoes, without leaving the comfort of your own home. You might be surprised to find someone on the other side of the country struggling with the same diabetes frustrations. You don't need to be a Web expert or even own your own computer. Most public libraries provide free Internet connections that you can use in half-hour sessions, just by signing in with your library card, which is also free. You can easily find plenty of resources via any Internet search engine by typing in the term "diabetes support" or something similar. See chapter 21 for a full guide of online diabetes resources.

Doctor Frustration

Many people with diabetes actually feel shunned by their own doctors. They feel they can't reach their doctor when needed, their phone calls are never returned, or from one appointment to the next, "The doctor didn't even remember who I was." On top of that, many patients often leave their appointments feeling deflated: the doctor's recommendations seem impossibly difficult, or depressing, or unhelpful once they've left the clinic and reentered the real world.

What you can do

It's definitely worth taking the time to find the right medical providers, because finding the right doctor can be like finding a friend. Only a doctor who understands your own unique learning style is going to be able to help you succeed.

Networking is always a good start: ask your friends, or ask at the local ADA chapter for a recommendation. Ask medical personnel with whom you already have a good relationship if they can recommend other professionals, rather than just picking names out of your insurance handbook based on convenient location. When you find people you like, stick with them. Keep your appointments.

And remember that simply believing "it's all the doctor's fault" is unproductive. This distracts you from what you need to do yourself. Quite a lot depends on how you approach your appointments. Keep in mind that *you* are the leader of your diabetes care team. Everyone else is there to support you. You'll get more out of your visits if you go in prepared with specific questions and action items. See chapter 3 for tips on managing the outcome of your own appointments.

Unsolicited and/or Wrong Advice

When you have diabetes, you'll find that people—loved ones and strangers alike—make a lot of exasperating comments. They say things like, "Are you sure you can eat that?" "No thanks? But I made this specially for you!" "Your blood sugar must be low—you need some insulin," or "My grandmother had diabetes and lost both legs and went blind." This kind of talk is not helpful to you!

What you can do

Simply asking people to stop making comments won't help, because they won't just stop cold turkey. What you can do is find a dispassionate moment (when everyone is calm), and say, "I know you're trying to be helpful, but you're not. So here are some things you *can* do to help me: *don't* ask if I can eat that. But help me ensure there's always some diet soda in the fridge . . ." and so on. It may be as simple as educating these people with print articles or printouts that debunk whatever misinformation they're relying on. Hopefully they'll come to better understand your reasons for your behavior, such as *why* eating a quick snack while a meal is cooking for an hour in the oven is necessary and will not spoil your dinner. Don't let your desire to "not make waves" or to please others keep you from working toward your essential health goals.

Make sure that what you're asking for is reasonable. On one hand, you may want to be treated like you're "normal," as in not having diabetes. Yet on the other hand, you need some understanding and appreciation of all the work and aggravation involved with this disease. So what *should* your friends and associates say and do to be supportive to you? Think about some things people did that were actually helpful, and keep those in mind to suggest at an appropriate moment.

The Supplies and Devices "Hassle Factor"

First, there's the hassle of filling and refilling numerous prescriptions, and then the never-ending hassle of continuously carrying and using them. For many people, the main frustration is obtaining their medications and dealing with the insurance, as in "Why does my pharmacy make me tell them that I have diabetes every month?"

In addition, there's the social hassle of worrying that your diabetes care routine may bother some observers. Some people have actually been told, "You can't test your blood here, right out in front of everyone." But the bathroom may be far away and totally inconvenient. This is not fair to you.

What you can do

In terms of prescriptions, it helps to get organized. If you're picking up your supplies at a local pharmacy, ask your doctor to help you synchronize the prescriptions so you only have to do one pickup per month. Also, review your supplies carefully each month so you don't run out too early—or you may need to ask your doctor to increase the quantities.

Also, find out whether your health plan covers a mail-order service for prescriptions. These generally offer three months' worth of supplies delivered to your doorstep, usually at cheaper co-pay rates. The convenience of phone-in or online renewals can be life-altering for anyone dependent on multiple prescriptions.

In terms of outsiders' reactions, it really is best to brief people in advance, so they're not surprised by your diabetes. For example, you can explain to your boss or coworkers what it is that you'll be doing with your meter, medications, or insulin injections. Assure them that while this is essential to your health, it's no big deal for them. It's just a tiny drop of blood you're drawing, and there's nothing remotely dangerous or contagious about it.

REAL PEOPLE:
SMALL FRUSTRATIONS CAN LOOM LARGE

MARCIE WAS A high-powered New York City account executive: supercompetent, fast moving, fast talking, and very successful. She took her diabetes seriously, and was also very skilled at mixing it in with her busy work and personal life. She had found a balance that worked for her, and maintained a strong Diabetes Health Account.

Yet one area of her diabetes care that Marcie had found *extremely frustrating* was dealing with the myriad of prescriptions she needed: two types of insulin, syringes, pen needles for her insulin pen, lots of glucose test strips, lancets, a large bottle of 81 mg baby aspirin, lisinopril, and a low dose of atorvastatin. Some, she ordered from a mail-order supply company (90-day supply packs), but she also liked to get her insulin locally, and this came in 30-day increments.

"I know that I deal daily with problems much more complicated than this, and I know how to do everything necessary, but still it just frustrates and depresses me—maybe more than it should, to have to do deal with the logistics of these multiple prescriptions all the time," she said.

In the end, it was Marcie's husband who created a solution. He was worried about her diabetes, and had wanted to do something helpful. But Marcie had told him that asking repeatedly about her food and blood glucose results was not helpful. What he did instead was take over the care of all her prescription needs: calling in for renewals, picking them up, and dealing with the necessary paperwork. None of this seemed like a big deal to him, but for Marcie, this intervention slashed her "diabetes frustration score" remarkably, putting her mentally into a much better place.

Try not to let all the small details of living with diabetes drain your energy; guide loved ones into doing something practical to help you, which can make you both feel more satisfied.

"I Never Get a Break"

Pending a cure, diabetes is forever, and it does require continuous attention, which can really grate on you. Wouldn't it be sweet to *just once* eat whatever you wanted without worrying about carbohydrate calculations and glucose monitoring?

National surveys actually show that the most prevalent "everyday frustration" with diabetes is in fact a sense of being overwhelmed: How do I stay on this blasted diet? How do I keep physical activity up? Do I really have to do all this sticking and testing? *Don't I ever get a break?*

What you can do

There are a couple of ways to ease up the pressure and give yourself a little "diabetes vacation" now and then. A dirty little secret is that most people already take regular breaks from their diabetes regimen, since no one can do it perfectly all the time. The trick is to recognize this, and find a way to take a "*safe* vacation" from your diabetes, according to Dr. William Polonsky, author of the very helpful book *Diabetes Burnout: What to Do When You Can't Take It Anymore* (ADA, November 1999).

An *unsafe* diabetes vacation is ignoring your diabetes for years. A *safe* vacation is one that you plan ahead, for example, taking a "day off" when you might eat a few taboo food choices or check your glucose less often than usual. This kind of break is okay as long as you're prepared for the consequences. You will need to recover from that day. And the break needs to be a one-time, conscious activity. You don't want to create an "on-" or "off-diet" mentality.

As we've emphasized in this book, it also helps to keep focused on your specific goals for the week or month. Are you trying to maintain an A1c level of 7.0, or reduce from a 10.0 to a 7.0? Are you trying to reduce your food intake? Or start an exercise program? If you can break down your diabetes care into palatable portions, you won't feel so overwhelmed by trying to be the "perfect diabetic" on every front at all times.

Understanding Stress

WE ALL USE the word *stress* a lot. You've surely heard about the ill effects of stress on both your psyche and your overall health. But do you know exactly how this applies to you?

Experiencing stress is more than having a busy lifestyle, because some people can juggle lots of activities and still stay calm. Stress is defined as a mentally or emotionally disruptive condition that occurs in response to adverse external influences—which can be physical, like injury or illness, or mental, like problems in your marriage, job, health, or finances.

In response, your body behaves as if it were under attack, usually characterized by increased heart rate, a rise in blood pressure, muscular tension, irritability, and depression. Your body prepares to take action with the so-called "fight-or-flight" response, causing many of your hormone levels to shoot up. Their net effect is to make a lot of stored energy—glucose and fat—available to cells. These cells are then primed to help the body get away from danger. In people with diabetes, the fight-or-flight response does not work well. Particularly in people with type 2 diabetes, stress hormones may directly alter glucose levels.

In addition, people who are under stress are focused on the thing that is causing their stress. They are much less likely to be focused on managing their diabetes. They may forget, or not have time to test their glucose levels. They may not follow their meal plan, or exercise as often as they should.

Short-term stress, the kind you get from taking a test or getting stuck in a traffic jam, is not generally the problem. It is the long-term sources of stress—things like working for a demanding boss or taking care of an aging parent—that can damage your health, because in your state of upset your body reacts to this nondangerous event as if it were a real threat. The stress hormones designed to deal with short-term danger stay turned on for a long time. Your body continues to pump out these hormones to no avail, and this can cause long-term high BG levels.

Your Personal Coping Style

Your coping style is how you deal with stress. What kind of attitude do you have when you're faced with a problem?

If you're pessimistic, you may say to yourself, "Things like this will always happen to me." Neither fighting nor fleeing is any help when the "enemy" is your own mind.

On the other hand, doctors everywhere note that patients who do best with their ailments are the optimistic ones. This is not because optimists are by nature "happy," but because optimism is really a copying style—a problem-solving approach. When a bad thing happens to an optimistic person, that person feels empowered to do something about it. Their conversations with themselves are practical and hopeful, as in, "Okay, now what can I do to make this situation better?"

IS STRESS AFFECTING YOUR BG LEVELS?

BEING STRESSED CAN have an effect on your daily BG levels, but the direct impact is relatively small. Where you run into trouble is the way most of us behave when we are stressed: we're much less likely to exercise, make healthy food choices, check BG levels with a glucose monitor, take medications on time, and perform the other tasks necessary for good diabetes care.

Stress distracts you from caring for yourself.

WHAT CAN YOU DO ABOUT IT?

Try some of these tactics:

- **Organize**—keep "to-do" lists, and be sure to prioritize. You can't do everything at once. Also, store your diabetes supplies at a handy central location.
- **Prepare**—plan ahead for the next day's activities, exercise, or meals, if possible. Use your BG records to anticipate highs or lows and how you will treat them.
- **Share your feelings**—don't try to go it alone. Sharing your feelings and frustrations is a great emotional release.
- **Go outdoors**—don't underestimate the benefits of fresh air, the sight of trees or ocean or other natural environments, and sunlight on your body and your state of mind. If you live in a city, find a quiet park where you can refresh your spirit.
- **Exercise**—physical activity is the best natural and portable stress-buster on the market.
- **Sleep**—without adequate sleep, your body functions at half-speed and tires out quickly. Most adults require about 8 hours a night, but a short 10- to 20-minute nap can be refreshing as well.
- **Become a volunteer**—it doesn't have to be health-related or a regular task, just something that takes your mind off your troubles while helping someone else achieve something good. You'll both benefit from the experience.

> • **Get professional help**—if your anxiety only increases, look for a mental health specialist to help you.

Recognizing Clinical Depression

TRUE DEPRESSION IS a serious problem, and people with diabetes are almost twice as likely to develop it as are other people. It's a vicious cycle because if you are depressed, diabetes can become a lot harder to handle and your BG levels are likely to rise. When your diabetes is out of control, this can make it even harder to escape depression.

So how do you define "depression"? How can you tell if you have it, versus simply feeling "down" or "blue"? This questionnaire, called the CES-D, was developed by the Center for Epidemiologic Studies. It is a useful tool for measuring your symptoms of depression.

ARE YOU EXPERIENCING DEPRESSION?

BELOW IS LIST of some ways you may have felt or behaved in the last week. Please indicate how often you felt this way by circling the appropriate number in the right-hand column.

Note that 0 means rarely; 1 means some of the time; 2 means occasionally; and 3 means most of the time.

During the past week:	**Rarely** or none of the time (less than 1 day)	**Some** or a little of the time (1–2 days)	**Occasionally** or a moderate amount (3–4 days)	**Most** or all of the time (5–7 days)
1. I was bothered by things that usually don't bother me.	0	1	2	3
2. I did not feel like eating; my appetite was poor.	0	1	2	3

During the past week:	Rarely or none of the time (less than 1 day)	Some or a little of the time (1–2 days)	Occasionally or a moderate amount (3–4 days)	Most or all of the time (5–7 days)
3. I felt that I could not shake off the blues even with help from my family or friends.	0	1	2	3
4. I felt I was just as good as other people.	0	1	2	3
5. I had trouble keeping my mind on what I was doing.	0	1	2	3
6. I felt depressed.	0	1	2	3
7. I felt that everything I did was an effort.	0	1	2	3
8. I felt hopeful about the future.	0	1	2	3
9. I thought my life had been a failure.	0	1	2	3
10. I felt fearful.	0	1	2	3
11. My sleep was restless.	0	1	2	3
12. I was happy.	0	1	2	3
13. I talked less than usual.	0	1	2	3
14. I felt lonely.	0	1	2	3
15. People were unfriendly.	0	1	2	3
16. I enjoyed life.	0	1	2	3
17. I had crying spells.	0	1	2	3
18. I felt sad.	0	1	2	3
19. I felt that people disliked me.	0	1	2	3
20. I could not get going.	0	1	2	3

SCORE

To get your score, follow these three steps:

Step 1. Take the sum of the numbers you circled in the right-hand columns, except for questions number 4, 8, 12, and 16.

Step 2. Add your total for those four questions, and subtract it from 16.

> **Step 3.** Then add the number you got in Step 2 to your orig-
> inal sum.
> **Step 4.** Review your score. Possible scores are 0-60. A score
> of 16 or more suggests depression.

We know from studies that about two-thirds of doctors fail to recognize depression. It may be that doctors don't ask the right questions, or patients just don't tell how they feel. In any case, if you think you fit the criteria for clinical depression, don't try to go it alone. And don't just wait around hoping it will go away. Instead, you should talk with your doctor as soon as possible and ask for a referral to a mental health professional. Research indicates that professional counseling, sometimes in combination with antidepressant medication, is a very effective treatment for depression.

As with diabetes, there is no one-size-fits-all treatment for depression. The strategy should be must be carefully worked out by a trained professional based on the circumstances of the individual and their family. Both psychotherapy, or "talking" therapy, and prescription antidepressant medications can be very effective.

But keep in mind that recovery from depression takes time. Antidepressant medications can take several weeks to work and may need to be combined with ongoing therapy. Not everyone responds to treatment in the same way. Prescriptions and dosing may need to be adjusted.

One of the biggest problems with depression is that it often recurs within individuals, so that they go through many cycles of depression and relative health. Doctors suspect that the more time a person spends depressed, the greater the risk for diabetic complications and death—a somber thought.

This is why it is vitally important to seek professional help if you are depressed—you need someone to intervene to help you stop the destructive cycle of recurrent depression.

Some Resources on Diabetes and Mood

Books

Psyching Out Diabetes: A Positive Approach to Your Negative Emotions by Dr. Richard Rubin, June Biermann, and Barbara Toohey (McGraw-Hill, November 1999).

Diabetes Burnout: What to Do When You Can't Take It Anymore by Dr. William Polonsky (American Diabetes Association, November 1999).

Zen and the Art of Diabetes Maintenance: A Complete Field Guide for Spiritual and Emotional Well-Being by Charles Creekmore (American Diabetes Association, April 2002).

Caring for the Diabetic Soul: Restoring Emotional Balance for Yourself and Your Family (American Diabetes Association, August 1997).

Meditations on Diabetes: Strengthening Your Spirit in Every Season by Catherine Feste (American Diabetes Association, February 1999).

365 Daily Meditations for People with Diabetes by Catherine Feste (American Diabetes Association, August 2004).

When You're a Parent with Diabetes by Kathryn Gregorio Palmer (Healthy Living Books, April 2006).

Programs

- Behavorial Diabetes Institute (www.behavioraldiabetes.org) —a newly established institute in San Diego offering group and individual seminars on feelings and motivation.
- Divabetic (www.divabetic.com)—diabetes coaching classes in New York, taking a bold, sassy approach to improving diabetes inspiration and motivation. Special focus on avoiding denial.

- Naomi Berrie Center in New York (http://nbdiabetes.org/patient_care/patient_family.html)—a forward-thinking family-based diabetes care program.
- Diabetes and Depression Laboratory, University of Ohio (http://www.psych.ohiou.edu/labs/degroot.html)—academic study and treatment programs.

20 Complementary and Alternative Medicine

Taking Charge of Your Health Is Good Medicine

IF YOU HAVE diabetes, and are reading this book, chances are good that you're already using some form of complementary medicine. Surveys have shown that over half of patients with diabetes use complementary medicines, for four common reasons:

- Wanting to make your own choices about your diabetes, rather than just being told what to take by your doctor
- A suspicion that traditional doctors avoid complementary medicine
- The belief that complementary medicine is more natural with fewer side effects
- The hope that the chosen form of complementary medicine is effective

Some people choose these substances to treat specific symptoms, while others are motivated by hope for a more general health improvement.

However you slice it, these are strong reasons for looking at complementary medicine—because they are indicative of a "take-charge" approach by the patient, which is very important in achieving good health results.

We know this because studies show that most people who use complementary medicine also make more use of "traditional" care than others, especially preventive care such as flu and pneumonia vaccines. And since complementary medicine choices are usually not suggested by your physician, selecting them means that you are actively involved in thinking about your own health and diabetes care.

We feel that the most successful diabetes care involves a natural, holistic approach. But we also know that everything included under the umbrella of complementary or "alternative" medicine is not equal: some types are useful, some can be harmful, and the effects of others may be neutral, except for cost. We hope to provide information here that will guide you in your choices.

Alternative Approaches and Their Value

Complementary medicine, sometimes called *alternative* or *holistic medicine*, can be a confusing area, and much of this confusion stems from trying to define it. One common definition is that it encompasses anything that is done outside of a traditional medical office, covering such disparate disciplines as nutritional counseling, yoga and tai chi, relaxation and meditation therapy, chiropractic care, acupuncture, vitamins, herbs, and bottled supplements.

Published reports confirm the wide variety of complementary medicines in use. A large telephone survey performed recently at Beth Israel Deaconess Hospital, in Boston, identified eighteen different types of complementary medicine, with 1 to 16 percent of the survey participants using each of the eighteen types.

For purposes of discussion, we have grouped these different types of therapy into four categories: (1) mind-body, (2) nutrition, (3) herbs and supplements, and (4) homeopathy and others. We will also be discussing their effectiveness, especially in light of the fact that one definition of alternative medicine is "a treatment that has not been proven by traditional methods." This is an awkward definition, actually implying that traditional methods of medical treatment cannot test or prove the effectiveness of alternative treatments. It also ignores the fact that some types of complementary medicine have actually been shown effective in traditional clinical trial methods.

But some claims cannot be tested in a straightforward way. If an herb claims to increase your energy, invigorate your immune system, or "promote health," there is really no way to clearly prove or disprove these statements, since it is difficult to measure energy, immune status, and general health. The makers of these "nutraceutical" products (a takeoff on the word *pharmaceutical*, with *nutrient* thrown in) have lobbied very aggressively for wide marketing rights. As a result, manufacturers of herbs and supplements can use phrases such as "increase," "invigorate," and especially "promote" without providing any real evidence of their products' effectiveness.

Many of these products do little more than make the manufacturers rich. However, we can easily measure effects on BG and A1c, so we know that some complementary or treatments are genuinely helpful in patients with diabetes.

Self-Help and the "Feel-Good Stuff"

Relaxation therapy, biofeedback, self-help groups, massage, self-prayer and prayer by others, hypnosis, and imagery

This group includes the most frequently used complementary medicine therapies, and some of the most effective. These approaches are also an example of the blurring of lines between traditional and complementary medicine, as classical clinical studies have shown the effectiveness of relaxation techniques (including meditation) and biofeedback on reducing blood pressure and lowering A1c. Self-help groups have been shown to be very effective for people with chronic diseases, and for diabetes in particular.

What's important here is the effectiveness, availability, low cost, and lack of side effects of these approaches. One study that underscored the effectiveness of relaxation therapy on improving diabetes control in teenagers was particularly eye opening, because it was the parents who received the therapy. (There's an idea for dealing with overly helpful family and friends; by getting them to "chill out," you may be able to improve your own bottom line.). The remaining therapies in this group have not been as well tested, but may have positive effects on your general mind-set and well-being, which is certainly valuable for your diabetes care.

Natural Medicines

Herbal medicine, dietary supplements, megavitamins, folk remedies

This is the most problematic group. A visit to a health food store such as Vitamin World or GNC will reveal an enormous number of herbs, vitamins, and mineral supplements that are touted to improve your diabetes. You can buy books written by PhDs and MDs that promote these products and seem to offer clinical documentation of their positive effects. You can even buy a copy of a well-known book titled *Reversing Diabetes*. (Why just treat it, when you can reverse it?) What should you make of these claims?

A 2003 project at Harvard Medical School reviewed published reports on forty-five different herbs and vitamins, and their effects on diabetes. Some of the studies suggested a positive effect, but in general the studies were too small, or the results were not repeatable, or they were poorly done. (See chapter 5 for details on what makes a scientific study credible.)

Several herbs and supplements are promising for helping diabetes treatment, including common spices like cinnamon, which appears to help keep BG levels in check. But none of these effects have been substantiated enough for us to recommend any particular supplements at present.

An additional concern with all of these "natural medicines," as opposed to treatments in the other three groups of complementary medicine, is that some vitamins and supplements are known to interfere with current FDA-approved medications, and most of them have not been tested for interactions with other medications, or for long-term side effects. In addition, there's some concern about variation in content, since there is no mandatory oversight or regulation on the purity or exact content of these substances. So you really don't know what you're taking.

Thus, our recommendation is to avoid complementary therapies in this group for the time being, even if they place what sound like very convincing ads in major periodicals or on television. Likewise, beware of Internet offers for a miracle cure—if there were one, why isn't diabetes already wiped out?

But, you may be asking, what if some of these therapies *are* effective, how would I know? The answer lies in the fact that treatments improving BG levels and A1c are easily identified, since these effects can be accurately measured. So if some supplement is effective, it won't be a secret for long.

Consider two examples: that fungal broth we mentioned as being developed in Japan is said to improve cholesterol, and an herb known as Goat's Rue or French Lilac is said to lower BG levels. In the first case, the substances in the fungal broth were purified and isolated, and a specific compound was found to have the cholesterol-lowering effect. This compound was further tested for side effects, and was then named lovastatin, the first of the statin medications to be discovered, and it is still used today. In a similar fashion, the components of French Lilac were identified, and one, named guanidine, was found to lower BG in animals. However, it was found to be too toxic for use in people. Further research produced biguanidines, which effectively lowered BG without toxicity. Today, one of these biguanides, called metformin, is the most commonly used medication for lowering BG in patients with type 2 diabetes.

Lovastatin and metformin are better treatments than the original fungal broth, or French Lilac. And because they are produced according to FDA guidelines, you are ensured consistent content and effect for every pill. If any of the abundant herbs and supplements currently being tested do prove to be consistently effective, you can rest assured that these results will be well publicized, and that the product will come to market in a big way.

What if the helpful compound is something as common as cinnamon, however? How could a pharmaceutical company make a profit off of a drug that it couldn't patent? The answer is that pharmaceutical companies are experts at making profits. They would have several paths available: identifying and patenting the active component in cinnamon, processing the cinnamon to a more potent form and marketing this as a tablet, or simply pushing their product as the "best" cinnamon. Does this sound ridiculous? Don't forget that a number of companies already make a nice profit by telling us that their water is better than other water.

In case you're still interested in exploring herbs and supplements and their relative value, a great resource is available from the National Diabetes Information Clearinghouse (NDIC) at http://diabetes.niddk.nih.gov/dm/pubs/alternativetherapies.

Special Diets

Commercial diets, lifestyle diet

"You are what you eat." This common tenet pays homage to the powerful effects of food in our lives. That food can effect how we feel and affect our health is common sense, and this common sense has been supported by clinical trials. Changes in the types of fat in your diet can improve your cholesterol; carbohydrate changes can improve your triglycerides; more fruits and vegetables can improve your blood pressure, and attention to amounts of carbohydrate will improve your A1c.

There is no single diet that is best for everyone, and *some* of the commercial and lifestyle diets can be a good fit with diabetes. By this we mean the likes of Weight Watchers, the South Beach

Diet, and Jennie Craig (although you may want to limit your commitment to buying their specially prepared foods).

In general, however, diets that require supplements to help you lose weight are not good choices. There are no supplements that help you to "burn off fat" or "change your metabolism." Keep in mind that since these products are classified as "nutritional," there is no authoritative oversight of their claims or content. Clinical studies of different diet plans have confirmed one commonsense fact: specific diet plans are difficult to maintain, and those that are more restrictive are more difficult to maintain. These studies have also confirmed that any weight loss associated with these diet plans is not due to any special quality of the diet (not the "ketosis" of the Atkin's diet, nor the balance of the Zone diet), but rather the weight loss results directly from eating fewer calories.

If you wish to choose a diet plan, choose one that is attractive to you in regard to the food types that it recommends, and choose one that you can imagine yourself continuing for years. One of the reasons that some diets (like the "Cabbage Soup Diet") remain popular is that you eat fewer calories at the outset and tend to lose weight quickly. But the weight comes back on almost as quickly when you stop the diet, because its very exclusivity makes it not sustainable. Then, when your weight returns, you feel that it is your fault for failing, not because the diet was unhelpful. Reasonable, sustainable changes in your eating habits are your goal here—not glamorous, but effective. One final comment: without the addition of regular physical activity, no diet is very helpful for weight loss.

Alternative Healing Treatments

Homeopathy, energy healing, aromatherapy, naturopathy, chiropractic treatments

Homeopathy is a prime example of the confusion surrounding some complementary therapies, starting with the fact that not many people know what this term actually means. Homeopathy is a system of alternative medicine that treats "like with like." The movement was founded in the 1700s in Germany, and entered the mainstream in the United States in the 1800s, where it soon became widespread and popular. Its founder, Dr. Hahnemann, developed a system for combating the adverse effects of various substances by prescribing a specific dilution of that very same substance—which would work to reverse the symptoms.

For example, if people drink too much coffee, they become nervous, shaky, and unable to sleep. The idea is that a specifically prepared homeopathic minute dilution of coffee in pure water will gently and promptly do away with these symptoms. If a toxic substance in a large dose causes nausea and vomiting, it is believed that an ill person suffering from the same or similar symptoms should take a homeopathic dilution of the toxic stuff in order to combat the symptoms.

Modern science seems to contradict this theory, however, since the dilutions are often so great that it is nearly impossible for *even a single molecule* of the original substance to remain in the prescribed dose. Nevertheless, a great many people feel they benefit from homeopathy. Why? There are several reasons. First, people often recover from a variety of maladies on their own just by believing that they are receiving a helpful treatment. This "placebo effect" is well documented in a number of areas, including common colds, and surgical and dental pain. In studies, patients receiving inactive substances (placebos) supposedly for pain control truly improved. That is, the patients not only "think" they are feeling better, but their bodies actually release potent compounds into their blood called *endorphins*, which are known to reduce pain.

Second is something called the "study effect": People who actively choose to take actions to improve their condition are likely to show some improvement, no matter what choice they make. This is believed to be a combination of the placebo effect and other conscious and subconscious forces taking place in these individuals, such as a strong determination to recover their health. This effect is often present in studies of type 2 diabetes, since patients taking part in these studies are "self-selected," meaning the type of people who step forward to participate in research studies are also likely to make helpful lifestyle changes, check their BG more often, and take their medications more regularly.

Homeopathic medications are ideal placeboes; they carry the promise of benefit, and generally have no side effects, except for a slight decrease in your finances if you overindulge.

By some accounts, the American Medical Association was formed in large part to counteract the growing popularity of homeopathy, and early members of the AMA were restricted from using homeopathic remedies. This antagonism has continued, to some extent, to the present day. Back in the 1800s, when it was introduced, homeopathy was probably an attractive alternative to primitive medical therapies of the day. The homeopathic treatments weren't likely to help you, but compared to the conventional medicine of the 1800s (which could also be very alcoholic, not to mention grisly with leeches and blood-lettings), they were less likely to harm you. Today, conventional medicine has come a long a way, and in the last fifty years in particular, the use of clinical trials has enabled people to make better decisions about treating complex diseases. Here's our recommendation: since the dilutions of many homeopathic remedies guarantee that they contain only water, we suggest that you save money, and just drink a healthy amount of ordinary water instead.

Energy healing (including the use of magnets), aromatherapy, naturopathy, and chiropractic treatments have shown no effects in improving glucose levels or A1c. All of these therapies are administered by well-meaning people who most probably believe that they can help your diabetes. Though you may feel a little better after using these treatments, keep in mind that they have no direct effect on your diabetes. If you are interested in trying one of these therapies to improve your relaxation and sense of well-being, consider massage therapy, which is quite enjoyable. Chiropractors, on the other hand, certainly can be helpful for some problems, but well-trained chiropractors are taught that there are some disease processes that aren't connected with the spine, and diabetes is one of those.

A Holistic Approach to Your Diabetes

THE LARGE NUMBER of available therapies—with varying degrees of proof concerning their effects—can seem quite confusing. Studies clearly show us the benefits of insulin, glucose-lowering medications such as sulfonylureas, metformin and TZDs, blood pressure and cardiovascular medications such as ACEIs, ARBs, and statins, but complementary approaches are harder to evaluate. Yet you might be wondering if a holistic approach to your health is still attractive? Aren't things that are natural better than things that are processed, or manufactured? The answer is yes; we agree completely that a natural, holistic approach is attractive.

But we take a more basic view than many of what is "natural." Eating foods rich in vitamin E and other nutrients is more natural than taking a capsule that contains 800 units of processed vitamin E. Not only is it more natural this way, but studies show that eating vitamin E-rich foods is beneficial, while taking 800 mg of vitamin E as a supplement is associated with a slightly increased chance of heart disease. Eating foods containing whole grains and fiber rather than more highly processed foods is natural, and again, studies show clear health benefits of eating them.

Interestingly, human insulin is perhaps one of the most natural diabetes treatments available. Patients now have access to insulin that is exactly the same as the insulin produced naturally by your body. On the other hand, no one can really provide ginseng that is as natural as something produced by your own body. It doesn't seem natural to take capsules or pills, even if they are sold in a "natural food store." Vitamins that have been "purified" into pills and herbs "concentrated" into supplement form are in essence no more natural than metformin, statins, or blood pressure medicines. But with the latter, we at least have the advantage of knowing that their production, purity and side effects are closely monitored, and that there are well-controlled studies demonstrating their effectiveness.

We would like to take this a step further and promote a holistic approach to your diabetes. But by holistic, we don't just mean anything labeled "natural." Rather, we mean looking specifically at all the parts of your life that effect and are affected by your diabetes. A holistic approach puts you at the center of the process, calling on you to make positive choices in a number of different areas that will improve your health. Physical activity is one of the central items here. As we've discussed, finding a way to maintain regular physical activity is not only helpful for controlling your A1c, but also improves your cholesterol and blood pressure, as well as your overall psyche.

Being knowledgeable about the food you eat is another central item. There's no underestimating the value of learning about food choices that will improve your health, and about how those food choices affect your mood and energy level. Reaching out to your family and loved ones, and involving them in your diabetes in useful ways, is also key to a holistic approach. The activity and food choices that help your health will also improve the general health of your family, and having them "on board" will make your life with diabetes easier. Reducing the stress in your life, including that resulting from diabetes, is extremely important, and has documented benefits. Plus, reducing your own stress is very likely to reduce the stress on those close to you.

ENJOYING A NATURAL, HOLISTIC APPROACH

HOLISTIC MEANS: recognizing that the emotional, mental, spiritual, and physical elements of each person comprise a system.

Holistic healing attempts to treat the whole person, concentrating on the cause of the illness as well as the symptoms.

Try applying these principles to your life with diabetes in a broad way:

- Use your muscles
- Eat whole foods, fruits, and vegetables
- Take an active role in your own medical care team
- Take the time to interact with your family, friends, colleagues, and neighbors in a positive way

Finally, don't forget to include your health-care team in this approach as well. As we've discussed in previous chapters, they are an essential part of your diabetes support system. You will need their positive input, especially at times when you may need to add medications to improve your A1c, blood pressure, cholesterol, or microalbumin. Use the information in this book to better understand the suggestions made by your health-care providers, and in some cases, even to suggest new additions to your regimen. Studies show that these common sense ideas are very effective for improving patients' lives.

ONCE AND FOR ALL: Finding out where you stand with your diabetes, and taking advantage of numerous treatment choices available, is your path to outliving diabetes with happiness and success.

21 Diabetes Resources:
Starting with the Internet

To SAY THERE'S no shortage of information available on diabetes
might be the understatement of the decade. In fact, the bigger
issue is how to sort through the abundance of news and information
you'll see coming at you once you've tuned in to the topic of diabetes.

How to Scour the Internet

WE START WITH the Internet because this is the best and easiest
place to find all sorts of resources, not just the online ones.

If you begin with popular search engines, such as Google,
Yahoo! or MSN, don't be put off by the literally millions of documents that come up for any diabetes topic. There are scores of diabetes resource lists, fact sheets, directories, FAQs, guidelines
documents and "About" pages. Not to mention the headlines and
health news sites and newsletters and home video guides . . .

Your best bet is to give some specific thought to what kind of site
you're searching for. Do you want to follow diabetes-related news stories regularly, or are you looking for a place to read personal stories
and connect with other people with diabetes? There are a number

of different "flavors" of Web sites dedicated to diabetes, offering everything from doling out headline news to offering a meeting place where visitors can interact. Nailing the right search term is a big help, as well. If you want the answer to a specific question, feed in as specific keywords as you can, such as "diabetic neuropathy" rather than "diabetes feet." On the other hand, if too few articles come up, you can broaden your search terms.

The sites of major diabetes-related organizations are good places to visit not only for their own information, but to find links to other, legitimate sites you might take ages to otherwise discover just by generally surfing the Web.

Since we can't possibly list *all* the interesting sites here, this chapter offers a quick introduction to your choices, with select samples from each category.

Sorting Your Favorite Informational Sites

A good place to start are the established advocacy groups like the American Diabetes Association (ADA) and the Juvenile Diabetes Research Foundation (JDRF). These sites include the ABCs of diabetes, along with a load of practical and research information. This category also includes other nonprofit organizations supporting research toward improved care, and an eventual cure.

From there, you may wish to check out the sites of some of the leading pharmaceutical companies, with their special diabetes pages and newsletters, to familiarize yourself with the treatments and products on offer. A third important category is medical news sites and news "aggregators" which pool top stories from a number of sources. Some examples from these categories are as follows:

Advocacy Groups (nonprofits) and Government Sources
- ADA—www.diabetes.org
- JDRF—www.jdrf.org
- Joslin Diabetes Center—www.joslin.org
- International Diabetes Federation—www.idf.org

- Canadian Diabetes Association—
  www.diabetes.ca/Section_Main/index.asp
- Children with Diabetes—www.childrenwithdiabetes.org
- Diabetes Research Institute—www.diabetesresearch.org
- The Iacocca Foundation—www.joinleenow.com
- Defeat Diabetes Foundation—www.defeatdiabetes.org
- National Diabetes Information Clearinghouse (part of
  the National Institutes of Health)—
  http://diabetes.niddk.nih.gov
- Food and Drug Administration—www.fda.gov/diabetes
- Insulin Pumpers—www.insulin-pumpers.org

Drug and Device Supply Companies

- Abbott Diabetes Care (glucose monitors, syringes,
  insulin pumps)—www.abbottdiabetes.com
- Animas Corp. (insulin pumps)—www.animascorp.com
- Ascensia (Bayer Diabetes Division; glucose monitors)—
  www.bayercarediabetes.com
- Aventis (Lantus long-acting insulin)—www.lantus.com
- BD Diabetes (glucose monitors, syringes, insulin injec-
  tion pens and needles)—www.bddiabetes.com
- Deltec Diabetes (Division of Smiths Medical; insulin
  pumps)—www.delteccozmo.com
- Eli Lilly & Co. (insulin)—www.lilly.com
- GlaxoSmith Klein (oral diabetes drugs)—
  www.gsk.com/yourhealth/diabetes.htm
- LifeScan (glucose monitors)—www.lifescan.com
- Medtronic Diabetes (insulin pumps)—
  www.minimed.com
- Novo Nordisk (insulin & injection devices)—
  www.novonordisk.com
- Keeping Well with Diabetes (a Novo Nordisk site)—
  www.kwwd.com/kwwd
- Pfizer (oral diabetes drugs, inhalable insulin)—
  www.pfizer.com

- Roche Diagnostics (Accu-Check glucose monitors)—
www.accu-chek.com/us/home.do
- Sanofi-Aventis (oral diabetes drugs)—
www.diabeteswatch.com

CONSIDER THE SOURCE

HOW CREDIBLE IS the information on any given Web site? Here are a few criteria to help you decide:

- Who's behind the site? Does the individual author or organization clearly identify themselves? If not, the "news source" may be just a front for selling some product line, or diverting Internet traffic to other advertisers.
- Does the site require you to register? There are a few legitimate media organizations (the *New York Times, Washington Post*) that call on readers to register, but many others are simply fishing for targets to add to their promotional e-mail lists. You should be able to read plenty of diabetes articles and gather information without inputting any personal information. If you can't access anything useful on the site without giving out your name and e-mail address, or even more, move on.
- Likewise, beware of any informational Web site that demands a membership fee. There are plenty of legitimate sites that you can access for free.
- Look for links and references. Any site sounding off on medical trends shouldn't be doing so in a vacuum, but should be referring to legitimate medical sources, such as academic journals.
- If the spelling and/or grammar of the site's information are atrocious, you really should wonder how much of the information there is accurate. Certainly, do not trust a site that cannot spell medical or pharmaceutical terms correctly.

- If doctors or other experts are quoted, you can Google these people's names to see whether any reports appear on the Web indicating they've made fraudulent claims or were involved in any malpractice suits.

- On sites run by organizations, look for the **HONCode** logo. This is an accreditation from the international, nonprofit Health on the Net Foundation (www.hon.ch), which serves as a watchdog for the credibility of medical and health Web sites.

- If the site contains links to or ads from really off-topic items (political or religious organizations, for instance), listen to your instincts and depart in favor of resources that are not trying to influence your values as well as your health.

- Time is a factor. Diabetes treatment and research is progressing so quickly that any information more than a few years old is in danger of being outdated. Look for sites that offer freshly updated material. You should be able to locate on the homepage or an "about us" page, when the organization and/or Web site originated, and when it was last updated.

- For security when making purchases online, never order any products from a site whose order form does not display the security "lock" in the bottom right of your screen, which stands for data encryption against hackers. Always print out a copy of your confirmed order form as a receipt and in case you have questions; don't assume the company will send you an instant e-mail to confirm your order. If no lock appears but the site seems genuine enough otherwise, phone their customer service department to relay your information to a live person. Or print out the order form, fill it in by hand, and mail it to them by regular post, keeping a copy for yourself. Never send critical information like credit card numbers via an e-mail message, which is not secure from hackers.

News Sites / Aggregators
- Diabetes Monitor—www.diabetesmonitor.com
- David Mendosa's Diabetes Directory—
  www.mendosa.com
- Medline Plus (provided by the National Institutes of
  Health and the National Library of Medicine)—
  www.nlm.nih.gov/medlineplus/diabetes.html
- WebMD—www.webmd.com/diseases_and_conditions/
  diabetes.htm
- About.com—www.diabetes.about.com/
- MedScape—www.medscape.com/diabetes
  endocrinology-home
- Topix Diabetes News—www.topix.net/health/diabetes
- MediCool Diabetes News—www.diabetesnews.com
- myDNA Diabetes Headlines—www.mydna.com/
  health/diabetes
- Yahoo Diabetes Health Center—
  www.health.yahoo.com/
  centers/diabetes
- Diabetes in Control (aimed at medical professionals)—
  www.diabetesincontrol.com/index.php

Find Your Connection via Online Communities

Online message boards, forums, and Web logs allow you to connect with other people in your shoes without leaving the comfort of your own home. You might be surprised to find someone on the other side of the country struggling with the same diabetes frustrations. Being able to toss out questions and ideas, and gain support and empathy is invaluable. No need to be a Web expert; you can easily find these resources via any Internet search engine by typing in the term "diabetes support" or "diabetes forum" or something similarly worded. (Don't be put off by some long, complicated Web addresses; these pages are generally easy to find from the main site as well.)

Message Boards / Forums
- ADA Message Boards—
  www.community.diabetes.org/n/pfx/forum.aspx?nav=ind
  ex&webtag=amdiabetesz
- dLife Community—www.dlife.com/forum
- vJoslin Discussion Baords—www.joslin.org/1861.asp
- DiabetesTalkFest—www.diabetestalkfest.com/forum
- Diabetes Forums—www.diabetesforums.com
- Dear Janis Message Board—
  www.websitetoolbox.com/tool/mb/dearjanis
- Diabetes Connect—www.diabetescommunity.com
- Diabetic Roundtable—
  www.s9.invisionfree.com/Diabetic_Round_Table/index.
  php?
- Diabetic Community—
  www.diabeticnetwork.com/community
- WebMD Type 2 Diabetic Support Group—
  www.boards.webmd.com/topic.asp?topic_id=1011
- WebMD Diabetes Management Discussion—
  www.boards.webmd.com/webx?50@871.QoCLaimJw5q.
  1@.5987f41a

Web Logs (Blogs)

This is a fairly new category of Web sites that is growing by leaps and bounds. Essentially, blogs are online journals that allow any individual to become a publisher on the Web. There are a few professional diabetes blogs run by media organizations, but most to date are maintained by patients wishing to share their lives and experiences with others. Readers can easily post comments to interact with the author and other readers on the site. Since blogs are still unfamiliar to many people, we've included a short description with each example below.

- **Diabetes Mine** (a gold mine of news, straight talk, and encouragement, from the author of this book, Amy Tenderich)—www.diabetesmine.com
- **The Diabetes Blog** (news and topics of interest presented by Weblogs Inc.)—www.thediabetesblog.com
- **Diabetes.blog.com** (discussion forums and personal anecdotes from an endocrinologist recently diagnosed with diabetes himself)—www.diabetes.blog.com
- **David Mendosa Diabetes Connections** (journalist David Mendosa reports on type 2 diabetes topics)—http://blogs.healthcentral.com/diabetes/david-mendosa/
- **Living with Diabetes** (a type 2 schoolteacher in Texas chronicles her life on an insulin pump)—www.kweaver.org/blog
- **Scott's Diabetes Journal** (a longtime type 1 diabetic in Minnesota shares his struggles and successes)—www.scotts-dblife.blogspot.com
- **Jo's Café** (Jo was diagnosed with type 2 diabetes in 2004)—www.joscafe.com
- **The Beautiful Diabetic** (a displaced Texan living in Oslo, Norway, and diagnosed with type 2 diabetes in June 2005)—www.thebeautifuldiabetic.blogspot.com
- **Noncompliant** (a working mother of two on managing her diabetes and her life at the same time)—www.noncompliant.blogspot.com
- **Diabetic Feed** (news and interviews, also offered via an audio broadcast (podcast) that can be downloaded onto a computer or MP3 player)—www.diabeticfeed.blogspot.com
- **The Diabetes OC** (online community site monitoring all known diabetes blogs to date)—www.diabetesoc.blogspot.com

BECOMING A BLOGGER

IF YOU FEEL you have something to share on a regular basis, you may wish to start your own Web log. It's easy. Here are a few of the best-known blogging "host software" providers to choose from:

- Blogger (www.blogger.com)—Google's proprietary software, free of charge and easy to use, but not ideal for more elaborate site designs
- Wordpress (www.wordpress.com)—another free blog service with an easy-to-use interface, recently upgraded with lots of handy features
- Typepad (www.sixapart.com/typepad)—a full-featured program from SixApart offering a variety of subscription levels with increasingly powerful design features
- Moveable Type (www.sixapart.com/movabletype)—also from SixApart, popular among bloggers who like to manipulate Web designs, formats, and functions—but you need some programming skills (or pay for an installation service) and your own Web host
- LiveJournal (www.sixapart.com/livejournal)—a community-based blogging system from the same company, offering quick and easy setup, but blogs often look more like forums or chat sessions than Web pages with structured content
- AOL Journals (http://peopleconnection.aol.com/journals/)—a free feature of the AOL service, easy to set up, but tends to restrict interaction with readers or other bloggers using different software

Discovering Print Publications and Local Resources

ANOTHER WAY TO use the Internet, of course, is to search for resources in the "real world." You can look up books, products, and even support groups and classes that might meet in your city. A number of diabetes magazines are available for reading online as well as at newsstands and via mail subscription. Again, we offer a list of some of the most prominent titles:

Magazines and Journals

- **Diabetes Forecast** (www.diabetes.org/diabetes forecast/back-issues.jsp)—a monthly magazine from the American Diabetes Association
- **Diabetes Voice** (www.diabetesvoice.org)—a monthly publication of the International Diabetes Foundation
- **Diabetes Health** (www.diabeteshealth.com)—the leading independent, investigative magazine for patients and medical providers
- **Diabetes Self-Management** (www.diabetes-self-mgmt.com) —an independent journal of practical "how-to" information for patients
- **Diabetes Care** (http://care.diabetesjournals.org)—an academic journal from the American Diabetes Association
- **Diabetic Mommy Online Magazine** (www.diabeticmommy.com)—a site for diabetic women who are pregnant, trying to conceive, or raising children
- **Diabetic Gourmet Online Magazine** (www.diabetic gourmet.com)—part of the Diabetic Connection network at www.diabeticnetwork.com/community
- **Diabetic Cooking Magazine** (www.diabeticcooking.com)— a monthly magazine focused solely on food management and dietary needs
- **Diabetic Living Magazine** (www.bhg.com)—a monthly glossy publication from *Better Homes & Gardens*
- **Diabetic Lifestyle Online Magazine** (www.diabetic-lifestyle.com)—an independent, Web-based magazine from two diabetic book authors
- **Diabetes Digest Magazines** (www.diabetesdigest.com)—a family of publications distributed free by pharmacies

around the United States, including Walgreens and
Wal-Mart

Groups and classes

You might not realize that informational classes and seminars are
offered around the country by community groups and diabetes supply companies for minimal or no entrance fees. This is a great way
to mix with other people with diabetes and learn something new
about achieving better control at the same time. These classes
cover the basics of diabetes causes and effects, glucose trends, carbohydrate counting, exercise strategies, preventing heart disease,
and much more.

Two examples of nationwide programs are:

- TCOYD (www.tcoyd.org)—this stands for Taking Control
  of Your Diabetes, a nonprofit group that offers full-day
  seminars around the country for a very modest entrance
  fee of around $35, including lunch
- Medtronic Diabetes Patient Information Event Series
  (www.minimed.com/events/intro)—check the company's Web site for classes planned in your area, free of
  charge

Finding classes and support groups specific to your own area is
as simple as a quick online search or calling your local hospital.
Some examples of great regional programs are:

- Divabetic (www.divabetic.com)—diabetes coaching
  classes in New York, taking a bold, sassy approach to
  improving diabetes care—with a current awareness cam-
  paign called "Denial's Not My Style"
- Behavorial Diabetes Institute (www.behavioraldiabetes.
  org)—a newly established institute in San Diego offering
  group and individual seminars on topics like "Feeling

Good Again" and "Discovering Your Own Motivation for
Managing Diabetes"

To assist you in your online search there are a number of useful "locator" sites to get you started:

- ADA Education Program Locator—
  www.diabetes.org/education/edustate2.asp?loc=x
- AADE (American Association of Diabetes Educators)—
  www.members.aadenet.org/scriptcontent/map.cfm
- dLife Support Group Locator—
  http://web4.dlife.com/dLife/do/
  ShowSupportGroupRecordSearch
- Ashley's Diabetes Information Center—
  www.elviradarknight.com/diabetes/supportgroups.html
- Defeat Diabetes Foundation—
  www.defeatdiabetes.org/support_groups.htm
- Cellscience Diabetes Charities & Support—
  http://cellscience.com/DIACharities.html

Where to Turn for Personalized Help

If you or someone you love is overwhelmed or undermotivated
far beyond the point of a good pep talk, there's still someplace to
turn. Clinics and medical groups across the country now offer top-
notch diabetes education and meal-planning programs that are *personalized* for each individual patient. These one-on-one sessions
with an educator or nutritionist help patients work out a treatment
plan that fits their own lifestyle, so they can experience success
rather than continuous feelings of failure.

You'll also do well to find out if your nearest major university
houses a diabetes center. Here you are sure to find cutting-edge
research and care, including great one-on-one "customized" assistance. People with diabetes a decade or so ago could only dream
of such help!

Appendix

Your Diabetes Health Account

Make copies of this table to fill in, update, and bring along with you to appointments with your doctor or educators. You may want to paste a copy on your refrigerator as well, to keep your health goals in plain view.

YOUR DIABETES HEALTH ACCOUNT

	A1c Target	Your A1c	Blood (BP) pressure Target	Your BP	LDL	Your LDL	HDL	Your HDL	Triglycerides	Your TriGl	Microalbumin (MA)	Your (MA)	Eye Exam	Your Eye exam
💰💰💰💰💰💰	≤ 6.5		≤ 120		≤ 80		≥ 55		≤ 80		≤ 30		No evidence of retinopathy	
💰💰💰💰	≤ 7.0		≤ 130		≤ 100		≥ 45		≤ 150		≤ 30		Minimal of retinopathy	
💰💰	≤ 8.0		≤ 135		≤ 120		< 45		≤ 250		≤ 40		Minimal of moderate	
💰	≤ 9.0		≤ 140		≤ 140				200-400		40-300		Pre-proliferative	
PAST DUE	> 9.0		> 140		> 140				> 400		> 300		Proliferative or macular edema	

Index

The Marlowe Diabetes Library

Good control is in your hands.

MARLOWE DIABETES LIBRARY titles are available from on-line and bricks-and-mortar retailers nationally. For more information about the Marlowe Diabetes Library or any of our books or authors, visit www.marlowepub.com/diabeteslibrary or e-mail us at goodcontrol@avalonpub.com

---

THE FIRST YEAR®—TYPE 2 DIABETES
An Essential Guide for the Newly Diagnosed, 2nd edition
Gretchen Becker I Foreword by Allison B. Goldfine, MD ■ $16.95

PREDIABETES
What You Need to Know to Keep Diabetes Away
Gretchen Becker I Foreword by Allison B. Goldfine, MD ■ $14.95

THE NEW GLUCOSE DIABETES REVOLUTION
**The Definitive Guide to Managing Diabetes and Prediabetes
Using the Glycemic Index**
Dr. Jennie Brand-Miller, Kaye Foster-Powell,
Dr. Stephen Colagiuri, Alan Barclay ■ $16.95
(Coming Spring 2007)

THE NEW GLUCOSE DIABETES REVOLUTION LOW GI GUIDE TO DIABETES
The Quick Reference Guide to Managing Diabetes Using the Glycemic Index
Dr. Jennie Brand-Miller and Kaye Foster-Powell with Johanna Burani ■ $6.95

THE 7 STEP DIABETES FITNESS PLAN
Living Well and Being Fit with Diabetes, No Matter Your Weight
Sheri R. Colberg, PhD I Foreword by Anne Peters, MD ■ $15.95